PRACTICE ISSUES
in Physical Therapy

Current Patterns and Future Directions

Jane Mathews MPH, PT

SLACK Incorporated, 6900 Grove Road, Thorofare, New Jersey 08086

SLACK International Book Distributors

Japan
  Igaku-Shoin, Ltd.
  Tokyo International P.O. Box 5063
  1-28-36 Hongo, Bunkyo-Ku
  Tokyo 113
  Japan

Canada
  McGraw-Hill Ryerson Limited
  300 Water Street
  Whitby, Ontario
  L1N 9B6

Australia
  McGraw-Hill Book Company
  4 Barcoo Street
  Roseville East 2069
  New South Wales
  Australia

United Kingdom
  McGraw-Hill Book Company
  Shoppenhangers Road
  Maidenhead, Berkshire SL6 2QL
  England

In all other regions throughout the world, SLACK professional reference books are available through offices and affiliates of McGraw-Hill, Inc. For the name and address of the office serving your area, please correspond to

McGraw-Hill, Inc.
Medical Publishing Group
Attn: International Marketing Director
1221 Avenue of the Americas —28th Floor
New York, NY 10020
(212)-512-3955 (phone)
(212)-512-4717 (fax)

Editorial Director: Cheryl D. Willoughby
Publisher: Harry C. Benson

Printed in the United States of America

Library of Congress Catalog Card Number: 86-04296

ISBN: 1-55642-006-4

Published by: SLACK Incorporated
           6900 Grove Road
           Thorofare, NJ 08086-9447

Last digit is print number: 10   9   8   7   6   5

Dedication

This book is dedicated to the many members who so willingly invest their time and effort serving as delegates in the American Physical Therapy Association (APTA) House of Delegates. Although the delegate constituency experiences a changeover of approximately one-third each year, there are many members who return as delegates for multiple years. They do so to confront the issues facing our profession and to set policy and position directions for the APTA.

I would be remiss in this dedication if I failed to include the House officers (i.e., speaker, vice-speaker and secretary) and staff whose joint efforts ensure the effective operation of the Association's democratic governance process.

This book, by no means, addresses the entire range of issues in Physical Therapy. However, it has the potential of serving as a cross-sectional information and education resource for present and future House delegates, members, and students who recognize the importance of being conversant in contemporary issues facing the profession of Physical Therapy.

Contents

Acknowledgments

I thank my spouse and colleague, Dr. John T. Gentry, for his continuing patience and support in all of my professional endeavors. He has consistently and persistently encouraged my professional activities, and serves as my most relentless critic. However, he does so in a manner that is unquestionably constructive. His strong value commitment to physical therapists, and their unique contributions to the health care industry, was firmly in place long before he met me. I truly appreciate that value commitment and can only hope that his longtime exposure to me has served to strengthen that appreciation and commitment.

Toward a Profession of Substance

In our evolution as a profession, we are at a critical crossroads. I believe that we have moved beyond our stages of adolescent rebellion and into our adulthood. Granted that those rebellions were absolutely necesssary and have resulted in the attainment of an independent accreditation program, direct access legislation in 21 states thus far, and the fruition of about 14 years of effort in planning and implementing mechanisms for formal Board Certification in six recognized physical therapy specialization areas. Those and many other efforts designed to advance the profession and enhance the quality of the services we provide were pathways laden with problems and barriers.

Recently, we have had a high measure of success in confronting directly some of those problems and barriers, not the least of which are the public's perceptions of our profession and the lack of awareness of the broad array of services we can provide. Our public relations campaign has helped immensely in improving the visibility of physical therapy as a major and essential component of the health care industry.

Our credibility, however, is still in need of vast improvement. It is time for us to launch concerted and intensified efforts to become a profession of substance. We must initiate activities that will help us to identify those elements that are solid and real in our profession as opposed to those that are superficial. The health care industry is about to sail into the 21st century and, in my perspective, physical therapy has one foot on the boarding ramp and the other foot on the dock. That is a most precarious position, and the decisions we make today have serious implications, not only for our future as a health care profession, but also for the extent to which we will be able to maintain and retain the professional achievements that we have made to date.

The following goals reflect the areas of activity that need immediate and intensified attention:

1. We must face the reality of the contemporary health care industry and the directions in which it is headed.

This is the reality. The total annual health care expenditures in the United States now exceed $500 billion, and this figure is projected to be in excess of $640 billion by 1990.

Great competition exists for those dollars. Currently, the health care industry is characterized by managed health care systems and megacorporations that are manifested as health maintenance organizations, preferred provider organizations, and a variety of joint-venture models. These managed systems rapidly and radically are changing the service delivery patterns and arrangements with which we have been accustomed for so long. Interestingly, but not surprisingly, the bulk of this change has occurred since 1983 and the advent of prospective payment systems.

This is the reality, also. Fee-for-service reimbursement, as we know it, is becoming obsolete rapidly. Directing time, energy, and resources to changing elements related to fee-for-service arrangements may constitute wasted energy. Physical therapy might be better served by focusing efforts and education on developing an understanding of other models of financial arrangements, such as group (not individual) capitation, so that physical therapists are in a better negotiating position with managed systems.

2. We must develop systems of accountability at all levels of APTA activity.

Managed health care systems and third-party payers are making it abundantly clear that they no longer are willing to relegate complete trust to the professional judgment of health care providers in respect to the nature and extent of services provided. More and more frequently, reimbursement claims are being denied retroactively with requests for substantive evidence that the services rendered have some measure of predictable cause-effect relationship with outcomes. In addition, third-party payer reliance on traditional forms of qualifications and credentialing, such as level of educational preparation and licensure, is waning rapidly. Their primary interests rest in seeking out providers who can achieve the desired functional outcomes quickly, efficiently, and with the least expenditure of resources. That is, managed health systems are interested primarily in the delivery of services that are cost-effective and in providers who evidence high productivity levels in the way in which services are delivered.

The APTA and its components have been engaged in quality assurance and assessment activities for many years. Some chapters have developed standards and guidelines to review and monitor physical therapy practice in their states. With some notable exceptions, however, many of these systems have not been implemented successfully because they depend on the voluntary participation of members. Some chapter officers have indicated to me that members do not make use of the systems that are operational. I am not certain that efforts to increase member utilization of the existing quality assurance systems are the best solution, but those efforts are necessary.

When we seek increased or more equitable benefit and reimbursement coverage from health insurance carriers, the first question usually asked is whether the provider group has an effect system of monitoring its services and its providers. In the meantime, most have claims review processes at several levels, and an increasng number of third-party payers are using physical therapists for second- and third-level claims review. Many of our colleagues involved in claims review, however, have to rely on their own experience and judgment in their review processes and lack reliable and valid criteria to use in review decisions. Furthermore, I suspect that few of our colleagues who function as claims reviewers for third-party payers realize the full nature and extent of their personal liability given the absence of reliable and valid criteria.

At the national level, we need to give direct attention to the development of valid and reliable criteria for claims review, and we need to mount efforts to train cadres of physical therapists who would be fully prepared to function as competent reviewers. Until we do that, third-party payers will rely on clerks, nurses, and administrative personnel to make criticial decisions that affect our professional services in a multitude of ways.

3. We must develop ways to be responsive to societal and public concerns in tangible ways.

As an example, the increased visibility obtained through our intensified public relations campaign will inevitably, if successful, increase the effective demand for physical therapy services. If we are in a supply situation that fails to meet that increased demand, however, our credibility with the public will be greatly diminished.

APTA survey data indicate a trend toward decreasing proportions of respondent members who are practicing in hospital settings. At the same time, the American Hospital Association is greatly concerned about what it perceives as the "shortage" of physical therapy personnel. Recently, I received a request from a voluntary health care agency for assistance in recruitment of physical therapy personnel. We must be responsive to those concerns, regardless of whether we agree with the perceptions of personnel shortages. In some of the practice settings where recruitment and retention appear to be particularly acute problems (eg, hospitals), those problems may be related more closely to factors in the practice environment than to shortages of physical therapists. Nevertheless, we must strive to assist those in practice environments and agencies and to help them understand ways in which they can make their practice settings more attractive to physical therapists.

If we are to be truly responsive to societal needs, we must remind ourselves that ours is a human service profession that evolved, and continues to evolve, around the unique services we can render to potential populations in need. If we lose sight of that mission, we will jeopardize all of the advances we have made as a human service profession.

4. We must place an increased emphasis on the importance of applied research and the resources allocated to it.

In no way does that statement diminish the importance and value of basic research. The demands, however, for substantiation of clinical intervention efficacy—particularly those from health insurance carriers—make it imperative that we address this need with urgency.

A study currently in process at Ohio University in Athens, Ohio, under the direction of Dr. Jeffrey Falkel, is a classic example of the type of research that is needed sorely. He is testing instrumentation and measurement that, if found to be effective, would provide greatly increased precision and predictability in the physiological effects of certain physical therapy interventions and modalities such as ultrasound. Many other similar investigative studies also are being conducted, and they are of critical importance.

In 1987, the APTA Board of Directors approved the distribution of a Request for Proposal that would result in data collection systems and studies that are designed to demonstrate the cost-effectiveness of physical therapy interventions. Substantiation of the cost-effectiveness of our services, as compared with those of other types of health care providers, is essential to our viability to negotiate in the contemporary health care marketplace.

5. We must be unified in our goals and the way in which we articulate those goals.

The growth of membership in the Association has resulted inevitably in a concomitant growth in the diversity of interests represented among the members. Dissension and differences of opinion expressed openly are healthy characteristics of any organization or group. We have a governance process that allows us to debate issues thoroughly at every level before taking final action in the House of Delegates. Debate should occur before the decision. When a decision has been made by a district, chapter, the Board of Directors, or the House of Delegates, we should articulate that decision in unity. Dissension occurring after major policy has been enacted, particularly when it occurs in public forums, can be a powerful barrier to achievement of our professional goals.

6. We must develop an improved capacity to be self-critical.

It has been said that no profession reaches full maturity as a profession of substance until it develops the capacity to be self-critical. The profession must foster an atmosphere in which uncomfortable questions can be asked. Otherwise, in the absence of such an atmosphere, we risk the danger of self-deception.

When others criticize us, those criticisms may or may not be valid. Nonetheless, we must be self-critical as we prepare our responses. It is not easy to raise uncomfortable questions, but they need to be raised. Gardner suggests that a certain amount of prudence is useful and uses the example of the Turkish proverb that says, "The man who tells the truth should have one foot in the stirrup."

7. If we desire to become a profession of substance, we must focus our energies and interests on what we intend to become and not on the achievements of the past.

It would seem to me that physical therapists are quite clear about what they want this profession to be and the changes necessary to achieve our goals. In sum, I have suggested that it is time to leave adolescent behaviors behind us and to proceed with the achievement of goals necessary to develop a profession of substance—a profession that has demonstrated its credibility and worth by differentiating its reality from its superficial appearance. Identifying our substance or reality is an essential and critical requirement if physical therapy is to be a viable and respected service in the contemporary and future health care industry.

Jane S. Mathews

CHAPTER 1

Issues and Trends in Physical Therapy Education

Geneva Richard Johnson, PhD, PT

"To everything there is a season, and a time to every purpose under heaven . . . "[1]

Physical therapy education is in a season of challenge, opportunity, and turmoil unmatched by any period in our history. Although no time has been free of the challenge of important issues, the continuing major changes that began in the past decade, in the whole of health care, have had an unsettling dimension not inherent in the challenges of other eras. Consequently, the decisions about education for the present and future must be based on careful examination and assessment of the significance of existing issues and those we can anticipate.

In 1918, when Mary McMillan opened the first educational program in the United States at Reed College, no future was envisioned for physical therapy beyond the cessation of hostilities and the rehabilitation of soldiers wounded in World War I. In fact, Vogel stated that "some physicians were skeptical, calling this program a 'passing fad.' They said it would soon be forgotten after the rehabilitation of the wounded had been accomplished."[2]

Ample evidence exists to show that physical therapy is not a "passing fad." Each year, approximately 4,000 graduates of educational programs in institutions in the United States enter the practice of physical therapy.[3] Programs may be offered at the baccalaureate degree, master's degree, or certificate level, or any combination of the three types. Candidates who hold a degree in a field other than physical therapy may elect to enter a program that offers a second baccalaureate degree, a master's degree, or a certificate.

The profession we practice today with such pride developed in response to identified needs in patient care. Yet without the vision, enthusiasm, self-lessness, and perseverance of the original physical therapists (called Reconstruction Aides in the World War I era), neither physical therapy education nor the practice would have survived. Physical therapists in those formative years readily transferred their knowledge and skills from care of the war wounded to care of those in a civilian population who suffered loss of physical function from trauma or disease.[4]

Physical therapists were resourceful in establishing a place for themselves in different environments. Their determination to maintain high standards of practice in the profession they created led to the formation of a national organization in 1921. Although originally named the American Women's Physical Therapeutic Association, the title was changed in 1922 to the American Physiotherapy Association, to allow qualified men to become members.[4]

Members of that young organization pledged themselves in the 1921 Constitution:

> to establish and maintain a professional and scientific standard for those engaged in the profession of Physical Therapeutics; to increase efficiency among its members by encouraging them to advanced study; to disseminate information by the distribution of medical literature and articles of professional interest . . . [5]

Advanced education for practitioners was a major purpose of the founders of physical therapy. By 1927, the Constitution also included as a purpose:

> to promote the science of physical therapy by cooperating in the establishment of standardized schools of physical therapy and encouraging scientific research in the profession . . . [6]

As further evidence of the importance placed on education by those intrepid members of the American Physiotherapy Association, a Committee on Education was given responsibility, in collaboration with Association officers, for setting a standard by which schools might form their curricula and state their entrance requirements. In 1930, a special committee was assigned the task of visiting all existing schools and determining their eligibility for approval according to the standards established by the American Physiotherapy Association.[6]

As early as 1928, the official publication of the American Physiotherapy Association, *The P.T. Review*, carried a listing of educational programs approved by the Association. Despite criticism from some quarters, the Association continued to serve as the accrediting body for physical therapy schools until 1933. According to Hazenhyer, in 1933:

> the Association was so anxious to maintain high educational standards in order to better serve the physicians and the patients, and so cognizant of its inadequacy to struggle with the complications, that it determined of its own violation, to appeal to the American Medical Association to take over the school situation.[7]

The cost of the process has been cited as a major reason for relinquishing control of accreditation. The resolution requesting that the AMA assume the function of accrediting, however, recommended that "the expense of such inspection (for accreditation) be borne by the school requesting the same.[7] The underlying reason for relinquishing control of that difficult process seems to have been the need to use an organization generally perceived as politically and financially powerful to carry out why may have been considered by a young organization as too burdensome a function for it to continue. Whatever the true reasons for divesting the Association of control of the accreditation function at that time, the issues surrounding physical therapy education and accreditation did not disappear.

The issues in education today are like those our founders faced in the first two decades of our history. For example, the quality of education, availability and qualification of faculty, admission requirements, educational standards, curriculum content, clinical education, accreditation of programs, applicants, finances, and organizational structure still are concerns. The issues selected for discussion in this chapter have been grouped under three major headings: nature of the profession, control of education, and preparation for practice.

Nature of the Profession

Definition

All issues in physical therapy education stem from the central one of identity. We must know who we are and what we want to become before we can plan and carry out educational programs to prepare physical therapists to function in an identified role.

In her 1975 McMillan Lecture, Hislop expressed the belief that physical therapy was then a profession in search of an identity. To end that dilemma, she proposed that physical therapy be defined as "a health profession that emphasizes the sciences of pathokinesiology and the application of therapeutic exercise for the prevention, evaluation, and treatment of human disorders."[8]

Other definitions have been proposed but none have had universal acceptance. The argument is that none cover the breadth of activities in which physical therapists are engaged or may undertake in the future. The same is true of the definitions used in the State and Commonwealth statues that regulate the practice of physical therapy. The specificity of the language in those definitions makes them unsuitable for general use.

Although the definition of physical therapy remains at issue, a philosophic statement adopted by the 1983 House of Delegates (HOD) of the American Physical Therapy Association provides a general description that may serve as a basis for arriving at a definition. According to the statement,

> physical therapy is a health profession whose primary purpose is the promotion of optimal human health and function through the application of scientific principles to prevent, identify, assess, correct, or alleviate acute or prolonged movement dysfunction. Physical therapy encompasses areas of specialized competence and includes the development of new principles and applications to more effectively meet existing and emerging health needs. Other professional activities that serve the purpose of physical therapy are research, education, consultation, and administration.[9]

This statement focuses on the primary concern of physical therapy; that is, the identification and the prevention, correction, or alleviation of acute or prolonged movement dysfunction. Implied, also, are the maintenance of function as an essential element in the prevention of dysfunction and the development of function as a normal process throughout life.

The brief statement characterizes physical therapy as a profession that has an obligation to use knowledge and skill for the welfare of society, to develop and apply new knowledge, and to prepare physical therapists for practice. Direction is provided in the statement, but no limits are set on the interpretation of service, research, and education in physical therapy.

If we accept movement dysfunction as our focus and pathokinesiology as the science of physical therapy, a specific definition may not be necessary. Because all of our interventions are aimed at enhancing movement in the whole body, broad interpretation of a philosophic statement will provide the latitude needed for removing artificial boundaries in the practice of physical therapy.

In that historic 1975 McMillan Lecture, Hislop also said, "if we will have the conviction and the courage to proclaim once and for all what physical therapy is and then act on it, the centrifugal forces generated will cast an ever lengthening shadow across the pages of human history."[8] The shadow has begun to form slowly.

Role

From the beginning of our history in the United States, the role of physical therapists has been a multifaceted one. As physical therapy has changed over the years, the role has expanded to include new responsibilities and functions.

In the present form of the role a physical therapist is a clinician, generalist; clinician, specialist; supervisor; manager; administrator; consultant; educator; and researcher. Because preparation for practice must attend to the entire role, each facet must be seen as a distinct area of practice. A physical therapist may assume responsibilities and functions that cut across the boundaries of two or more seemingly discreet facets. But in all facets of the role, a physical therapist is expected to be an advocate for the patient and family; a political activist on behalf of the public and the profession; a marketer of physical therapy services; a representative to community organizations; a fund raiser for needs in service, research, and education; an active participant in professional organizations; a continuing learner; and a contributor to new knowledge.

The issues related to the definition of physical therapy and the role of its practitioners clearly are interdependent. The role will evolve in relation to a dynamic definition that describes the potential scope and emphasis of the profession. To prepare physical therapists who are capable of practicing today and, at the same time, creating our future, educators must rely on a definition for guidance and direction in developing curricula.

Establishing a definition of physical therapy, therefore, is a critical issue. Modifying that definition to reflect changes in professional practice is equally critical to the continued development of a caring yet scientific profession that serves the health care needs of society around the world.

Control of Education

Physical therapy is gaining recognition as a profession through the gradual but steady movement toward autonomy in practice; the acquisition of social rewards such as salary, prestige, and privilege; an extended period of academic preparation to allow mastery of a large body of knowledge; and development of new knowledge through research. Although all physical therapists must be licensed to practice, which is a common trait of professionalism, some statues are so restrictive that they serve the welfare of neither the public nor the practitioners.

Describing the attributes of a profession, Goode made a distinction between the characteristics of a profession and the traits of professionalism. Goode states that "the core characteristics are service orientation and a body of theoretical knowledge."[10] Sussman added, "with autonomy of the work group as a by-product."[11]

In elaborating on the traits of professionalism, Sussman states that:

> the profession, through a self-organized collectivity identified as an association or society, determines standards of training and education for tasks and professional roles. The intended outcome is rededication and reinforcement of the service orientation, mastery of new knowledge for maintaining professional competence over time, and further division of labor which supports the rationale for autonomy.[11]

Control of the education that prepares individuals for the practice of a profession is at once a right and a responsibility of that profession. But educational programs are housed in institutions and, therefore, are subject to both internal and external controls. Both types of control are core issues and exert strong influence on the operation of an educational unit.

Internal Controls

Internal controls include the mission of the institution offering an educational program in physical therapy; the placement of the program within the organizational structure of the institution; and the availability and distribution of financial and other resources.

Mission

The primary internal control of an educational program in physical therapy is directed by the mission of the institution that houses the program. Every public and private institution of higher education was created to fulfill a specific mission. That mission dictates the educational emphasis of the institution, the population to be served, the operation of the institution, and the use of available resources.

In the past two decades, the mission of a large number of institutions seems to have been the determining factor in the establishment of a record number of educational programs in physical therapy. Accredited programs were offered in 47 institutions in 1969. Between 1970 and 1979, 30 additional institutions received accreditation for new programs, and another 32 were added between 1980 and 1987. Baccalaureate degree or certificate programs were initiated in 56 of the 62 new institutions offering programs, and 6 institutions opened programs at the master's level.[12,13]

During the same period of 17 years, two of those new baccalaureate degree programs were discontinued and two master's degree programs accredited prior to 1970 were closed, one at Case Western Reserve University in 1971 and the other at Stanford University in 1985. In 1981, the baccalaureate degree and certificate programs at the University of Pennsylvania also were closed.[12]

The reasons cited for discontinuance of a program usually include statements such as the cost of operation exceeds resources available to the program; the program is not central to the mission of the institution like those, for example, in mathematics, english, and biology; and professional education is inappropriate in the undergraduate liberal arts milieu of the university. Other reasons may be advanced but the most telling is the high cost of operation. Despite the fact that the known cost of operation is high, at least 14 new programs presently are in various stages of development.

Establishment of an educational program is a public proclamation of the value of the discipline to the institution and to those it serves, namely the students, the community at large, and the profession. An issue of grave concern is the rapid and continuing proliferation of programs without the development of appropriate financial resources and with an acknowledged acute shortage of qualified faculty. The quality of education, and consequently the competence of practitioners, is at stake.

The mission of an institution is the major controlling internal force for any educational program. An examination of the mission statement of institutions currently offering programs in physical therapy could raise serious questions about motives for continuing a program without sufficient funds to support an adequate number of faculty to teach and participate in research and clinical practice; provide physical facilities for teaching, research, and general operations; purchase or replace equipment for teaching and research; and supply materials and staff to support the faculty in teaching and research.

Organizational Structure

In order of priority as an internal control, the placement of the educational unit within the organizational structure of the institution barely ranks second to the mission in importance. By that placement, the administrator of the institution makes another public statement about the relative value of the unit. The placement establishes the titles of the unit and the academic administrator clarifies the administrative channels open to the academic administrator, and indicates clearly who will speak for physical therapy to the ultimate decision-makers in the institution.

In June 1986, the Department of Education of the APTA reported that of the institutions with programs, 54% had located them administratively in schools of allied health and 15% in schools of medicine.[3] In those settings, the educational unit is designated as a department, a division, a program, or a curriculum, and the title of the academic administrator may be director, head, or chair. The remaining 31% of the programs have various organizational placements and titles within their parent institutions; only four of those programs are designated as schools of physical therapy, and only two of those are administered by deans.

Without question, physical therapy has limited recognition in many institutions. A unit that is organized as a division, within a department, within a school, within the university, has little claim to visibility or power. The academic administrator lacks direct access to the ultimate decision-makers on policies that affect the quality and operation of the unit. Consequently, physical therapy education may have difficulty flourishing in an environment where the academic administrator is not an active, direct, and equal participant in all decisions that affect the welfare and operation of the program.

Administrative Support

Administrative support is essential to the development of an educational program of high quality. When the policy and decision-makers in an institution elect to organize and operate an educational program, the assumption is that a program of excellence will be created. A further assumption is that the necessary resources of the institution will be available to nurture and sustain that program in the growth to excellence.

If those assumptions are accurate, administrative support will be demonstrated by the following:

● Placement of the educational unit in a position of strength within the organization.

● Appointment of a physical therapist with academic qualifications and experience to organize a curriculum with the assistance of consultants and faculty members; recruit and recommend the appointment of a faculty; purchase equipment and materials for the teaching-learning process; direct preparation for the on-site visits for accreditation; assist in the development of a faculty research program; and develop a program for the acquisition of funds to support the program.

● Allocation of adequate funds to recruit and appoint qualified faculty and staff; employ consultants to assist in curriculum development; equip the educational unit for the teaching-learning process and a research program; arrange for sites for clinical education and the selection of a clinical faculty; develop library and teaching- learning materials; and prepare for the on-site visits for accreditation.

● Assignment of sufficient space for classrooms and teaching and research laboratories; storage; independent study area, lounges, and locker rooms for students; and offices for faculty and staff.

● Establishment of a development program aimed at acquiring funds for the needs of the educational unit; for example, general operations, special projects, endowed chairs, construction, and loans, scholarships and fellowships for students.

● Commitment to the continuing allocation of sufficient financial and other resources to develop and nurture the maintenance and growth of a program of excellence.

Establishing and maintaining an educational program in physical therapy may be a function of the mission of an institution. If administrative support is in question on any item cited above, however, that mission deserves careful review by the policy and decision-makers who must justify the establishment and continuation of any educational program within the institution.

Financial and Other Resources

Another strong internal control that regulates the operation and quality of an educational program is the allocation of the financial and other resources necessary for the development and growth of the unit. The quality of a program rests, in large measure, on the commitment of sufficient financial resources to attract and retain faculty members who are eligible for appointment and advancement in the university; to develop and execute a plan that promotes the growth and development of each faculty member; to acquire suitable teaching-learning materials; to equip and maintain classrooms and teaching laboratories; to equip and maintain research laboratories; to employ office personnel and teaching and research assistants for the faculty; to equip and maintain offices for the faculty and the office personnel; to develop a program of clinical education; to recruit and select students with potential for achieving the goals of the educational program; and to award scholarships, loans, and fellowships to students.

In many institutions, the cost of financing physical therapy education has risen sharply in the last decade. Much of the increase can be attributed to salaries for the faculty. To attract qualified faculty members, institutions have been forced to offer salaries and benefits that are comparable to the lucrative opportunities in clinical practice. Because choices in physical therapy education and practice are abundant, potential faculty members can negotiate for concessions, such as opportunities to develop their own research, establish a clinical practice, and continue their personal and professional growth.

The rising costs of education usually cannot be offset by external funding. Major gifts for operation and endowment are rare in physical therapy education. In most institutions, little emphasis has been placed on raising funds for physical therapy from the private sector. Although individual physical therapists have received funds for research from outside sources, including the federal government, a majority of the educational programs must operate soley on funds allocated by their institutions.

As leaders in education, academic administrators must become adept in securing external private and public funds for education, research, and other activities. To acquire finesse in approaching donors who are able to make substantial contributions, academic administrators, faculty members and students need assistance and guidance from experts in public relations and development who are either within the institution or the community.

Physical therapy in a health care profession that largely is unknown to the general public. Through an organized, concentrated development program, the public can be informed of the importance of supporting this unique health care profession and told how recipients benefit from the services of caring, concerned, competent practitioners. Promoting the profession to potential donors will not be difficult but does necessitate careful planning.

Equally important is the interest of administrators in mounting an aggressive campaign to attract funds for education and research.

The resources of institutions vary in number, type and quality. The ability of an institution to provide financial and other resources for physical therapy education should be examined under the harshest light. The cost of the program may exceed the perceived benefits to the institution, the students, the community, and the profession.

External Controls

External controls, whether subtle or overt, exert strong influence on decisions made by administrators within an institution and in an educational program in physical therapy. Those controls are not subject to any power the institution holds and cannot be ignored without consequence to the institution, the program, the students, and graduates. Those outside forces most likely to shape the decisions related to physical therapy education include programmatic accreditation, changes in the profession, changes in society, and availability of qualified faculty members and students.

Accreditation

The most direct and the strongest external control comes from the requirements for accreditation of educational programs by the Commission on Accreditation in Physical Therapy Education of the APTA. The standards used by the commission to judge all educational programs are determined by the APTA HOD, which is the representative and policy making body.

Accreditation as a voluntary and salutory process for assuring acceptable quality in education is not at issue. However, control of the process of accreditation and who should have the undisputed right to establish the standards for education do remain at issue.

A major change in the direction of physical therapy education occurred in June, 1979, when the HOD of the APTA established a policy requiring a postbaccalaureate degree as the entry level education for the physical therapist. In the same policy statement, the HOD fixed December 31, 1990, as the time of compliance with the policy.[14] Several efforts to rescind that policy have been unsuccessful, and in 1986 the HOD confirmed, without dissent, its intent to maintain the policy.[15]

Unanimous acceptance of the policy that the educational program offered in physical therapy must result in the award of a postbaccalaureate degree left no doubt about the need to prepare new standards of education for use in the future. To be current, standards must reflect the changes in demands made on a profession and the expectations of its practitioners.

Several drafts of new standards have been prepared and widely circulated by the APTA Task Force to revise standards for accreditation. Educators, clinicians, and researchers in physical therapy have been urged to present their comments in writing and at public hearings. Representatives of the larger community of interests (eg, officials in institutions and public agencies; members of committees, councils, and boards of the APTA; and representatives of organizations) have been invited and strongly encouraged to present their comments at the public hearings held in several convenient geographic locations throughout the country. The task force is scheduled to present a final draft for action to the 1990 HOD of the APTA.

The obvious link between the standards of education and the requirement for postbaccalaureate degree education for the physical therapist has caused administrators in some institutions and in some state agencies on higher education to threaten to withdraw from the national accreditation process. Some of them propose to establish a legal process for accreditation of physical therapy educational programs in their own states. Some have charged that physical therapists are self-serving, seeking aggrandizement at the expense of the public they purport to serve.

Some administrators question the right of the APTA to establish the postbaccalaureate degree as the required level of education. Their argument is that the right to establish the degree level rests with the institution awarding the degree. The 1979 policy statement, however, does not name the degree but merely states that the program offered must result in the award of a postbaccalaureate degree.[14]

Another facet of the issue on accreditation has been introduced by administrators who would eliminate programmatic accreditation altogether in favor of institutional accreditation. Accrediting agencies for the professions would be dissolved. If that plan were accepted, the public and professional communities would be expected to acknowledge institutional accreditation as the only criterion for quality control of education for professions such as dentistry, engineering, law, medicine, nursing, pharmacy, physical therapy, social work, speech pathology and audiology, and veterinary medicine.

Programmatic accreditation is an issue for other health professionals as well as physical therapists. No group is apt to relinquish the right without a struggle. The danger exists that selected professions may be permitted to maintain an accreditation function while others are not. That kind of discrimination could erode the quality of health care nationally by eliminating common standards for all educational institutions offering a program in any health care field.

Changes in the Profession

Since the introduction of physical therapy in the United States in the early part of the twentieth century, the profession has progressed steadily in the creation and acquisition of knowledge to substantiate the basis for practice in the development of skills in evaluation and treatment of movement dysfunction; and in concern for the total well-being of patients and clients of all ages.

Evolving Role of the Physical Therapist. The role of the physical therapist is evolving and can be described as fluid. All physical therapists, regardless of title or position, function in multiple capacities, shifting from one to another as the situation demands. For example, the clinician serves as a teacher, a supervisor, a negotiator, a clinician researcher, an advocate, and a business administrator. Physical therapists in other positions not only share those functions but may assume additional ones as well.

In 1958, Hislop and Worthingham reported that the annual attrition rate in physical therapy was 7%.[16] Gwyer's study of a stratified random sample of all 1972 graduates showed a 2% attrition for that group 11 years later.[17] Other studies do not report the attrition but the percentage of those who are still in practice 10 to 24 years after graduation.

Blood found that 95% of the graduates from Stanford University between 1970 and 1980 were in active practice.[18] Eighty-eight percent of graduates from Marquette University between 1956 and 1980 continued to practice.[19] Results of a 1983 study showed that 75% of Case Western Reserve University graduates from 1962 through 1971 were employed in physical therapy.[20] Hageman reported employment in physical therapy for 91% of the 1972 to 1985 graduates from the University of Nebraska.[21]

No generalization can be made from the findings cited except for the graduates of 1972. Nevertheless, the other studies are representative of all of the graduates of those four programs and cover the years from 1956 through 1985. A trend may be developing toward a longer total period of employment, whether it is continuous or interrupted.

Specialization. Although specialization has been a reality since the early days of physical therapy, no formal recognition was given to specialists by the profession until the Board of Certification of Advanced Clinical Competencies was formed by the APTA. That board has given rise so far to the development of specific specialty boards for certification in cardiopulmonary, neurologic, orthopedic, clinical electrophysiology, sports, and pediatric physical therapy.[22] Today, certification in any one of those specialties is a coveted achievement.

Technology. The introduction of technology into service environments has given the physical therapist tools with which to make accurate measurements of a patient's or client's physical status, to monitor and record responses to evaluation and treatment, and to analyze the results of evaluation and treatment. The computer can process data collected on patients, the outcomes of care, and the utilization of personnel, space, equipment, supplies, and time. In addition, the computer can schedule patients, personnel, and equipment; record the status of patients; and prepare bills and monthly and annual reports.

Research. Research by physical therapists has been a factor in creating changes in practice. Through research, the practitioner has been supplied with a rational basis for selecting certain physical therapy procedures for a particular patient. Research is laying the foundation on which to base clinical decisions.

Continuing Education. Continuing education has grown apace in the past decade and has been a major source of change in physical therapy practice. Armed with new knowledge from research and with skills acquired in continuing education courses, physical therapists have influenced change in practice by incorporating different approaches to patient care into their own practices.

Practice Sites. Practice has changed significantly as more physical therapists have chosen employment outside the acute hospital setting. A 1983 study showed that only 42% of all practitioners were in hospital settings while the remainder were in less restricted employment environments, such as private practice, community agencies, outpatient services, public or special schools, universities or colleges, sports facilities, or rehabilitation facilities.[23]

Legislation. Another source of change in practice has been the enactment of legislation permitting the public to have direct access to physical therapy services. To date, physical therapists in twenty-one states have achieved that measure of independence in practice.[24]

Changes in the practice of physical therapy are continuous. The pressures for change come from such sources as practitioners, the public, the state and federal governments, and organizations like the American Hospital Association. The future of physical therapy depends on how the profession responds to the pressure from any source.

Changes in the practice of physical therapy are a powerful external control that cannot be denied by the faculty of an educational program. To prepare a physical therapist for practice in the present and the future, administrators within the institution and in the educational program must be alert to the changes in practice as they occur and to the implications of those changes for the educational program.

Changes in Society

Prior to planning a curriculum in physical therapy, the needs of society should be explored carefully. Events of the past two decades have altered society in the United States.

Population Characteristics. The population of the United States increased from 203,302,031 at the time of the 1970 census to 226,545,805 in 1980.[25] That information is useful, but the features of the population that are important to note for physical therapy education are the distribution by age, sex, language, ethnic origin, geographic location, and place of residence.

Immigrants are encouraged to retain their native tongues and cultures. The United States is no longer a "melting pot" where English is the language of communication for all citizens, but is not a polyglot nation.

The number of adults beyond 60 years exceeds that of youth between the ages of 10 and 19 years by approximately 5,000,000; a majority of those older adults are women.[25] The problems of women differ from those of men. The needs of older adults differ from those of children, adolescents, and adults of other ages.

A large number of people are clustered in major population centers throughout the nation. A majority of the people, however, live in small cities and in rural areas of the country. The needs of people in cities differ from those in less populated areas. Additionally, the people who live in nursing homes, extended care facilities and retirement communities or facilities have needs that differ from patients who are in hospitals.

Emphasis on Fitness. A segment of society has invested in a lifestyle that emphasizes longevity and maintenance of a healthy body and mind. Prevention of injury or disease, continued development of the body and mind, and maintenance of strength, flexibility and endurance are important aspects of fitness throughout the life span. An equal emphasis in physical therapy education must be placed on prevention, development, and maintenance, as well as on the traditional aspects of restoration.

Concern for the Health of Peoples in Other Nations. Television has presented the impoverished, unhealthy condition of people in many other nations. Although a nation may be less deprived in natural resources, the lack of sufficient health care facilities and personnel to provide care may be a serious deterrent to health of that nation. Supplying funds and medicine is a humanitarian act. Supplying health care professionals to teach and treat will have a lasting effect.

The needs of society represent a major external control to which the institution must attend. The mission of most institutions dedicates the efforts of administrators and faculty members to meeting the needs of the segment of society they are obliged to serve.

Availability of Qualified Faculty Members

In November 1985, the APTA Board of Directors received the Report of the *Task Force on Faculty Shortage in Physical Therapy.* The report dealt with causes for the shortage and remedies to alleviate the problem.

The task force reported that in the Fall of 1984, administrators in 102 entry-level programs claimed a need for an additional 152 faculty positions to carry out the existing programs. They estimated a need to fill an additional 150 positions before postbaccalaureate degree programs could be initiated.[26]

Programs in 114 institutions in the United States now are in full operation[27] and others are scheduled for an on-site visit for accreditation in coming months. At least 10 other institutions are known to be developing programs.[28]

The shortage of qualified faculty members has serious implications. From the statements made by academic administrators in 1984, the shortage could be expected to rank high as an external control of education. Without sufficient faculty, the move to the postbaccalaureate degree may be difficult for some programs.

Preparation for Practice

From the time of the first human beings, physical measures have been available to use for healing, relieving pain, and increasing strength and endurance. Determining why and when to use those measures has become the science of physical therapy; how to use them, the art.

In the past two decades, advances in physical therapy practice, research, and education have paralleled those in other health professions. That is to say, phenomenal advances have occurred in selected areas and virtually none in other important areas. Despite real or assumed barriers, the leaders in service, research, and education have advanced the profession.

Physical therapy is not known or understood universally, as are medicine, nursing, and dentistry. That lack of understanding poses both advantages and some severe disadvantages. A disadvantage, for example, is that thousands of highly able and competent physical therapists are prevented from making their services directly available to the public because of antiquated, restrictive legislation throughout most of the United States.

Individuals seeking physical therapy services must pay a financial penalty because treatment of a physical therapist cannot be initiated without a referral from a physician or other designated, licensed, health care practitioner. The physical therapist has no choice but to exact that penalty. Even in those states that give the public direct access to physical therapy services, the financial penalty remains. Because third party payers refuse to reimburse their clients unless services are authorized by a physician or other designated, licensed practitioner, the inevitable conclusion is that physical therapy has not achieved acceptance as a profession.

Among the distinct advantages of being relatively unknown is that any undesirable stereotype of physical therapy is limited and can be overcome. Physical therapists still have the freedom for a short time to determine what the practice of physical therapy will be and, therefore, what the preparation for that practice will be like.

Although the current demand for physical therapists is high and is expected to increase 87% by the year 2000,[29] the nature of physical therapy practice and preparation for that practice are unsettled. That is an understatement of enormous magnitude. Physical therapy, even in its present status, is in real jeopardy of extinction. If third party payers, including state and federal agencies that write and enforce regulations purported to interpret the intent of legislation, continue to inhibit direct access to physical therapy services by discriminatory control of reimbursement, physical therapy will not be accorded professional status and will decline. The future of physical therapy lies in the decision made between the two forms preparation for practice can take—training or education.

Training is designed to meet immediate needs and is task oriented. Knowledge and skills acquired are specific to the tasks to be performed. Training implies that the performance of the graduate of the program will be monitored while an assigned task is in progress. The performance is evaluated against established criteria. The graduates are not expected or encouraged to make independent decisions.

Education is designed to instill in the learner the knowledge, principles, values, and skills that will be useful in identifying and solving problems in the present and in the future. The graduate is expected to make independent decisions, take action, and accept responsibility for the outcomes of decisions and actions.

If the preparation for practice is to come from training, the move toward postbaccalaureate degree preparation can be shelved. On the other hand, if education is to stand as the means of preparation for practice, the nature of that education becomes the most important issue facing the leaders and decision-makers today.

The level of educational preparation is linked closely to public recognition and acceptance of physical therapy as a profession. In 1979, when the HOD of the APTA resolved that all educational programs in physical therapy be at the postbaccalaureate degree level, omission of the degree to be awarded was deliberate. Some educational planners in physical therapy automatically assumed that the next level beyond the baccalaureate degree must be a master's degree. Clearly, that is not the model used by autonomous health care professions such as medicine, dentistry, and podiatry. All of those professions award a doctorate for satisfactory completion of postbaccalaureate education designed to prepare clinicians.

The future of physical therapy as an autonomous profession rests on its practitioners' educational preparation, the physical therapists' ability and willingness to assume responsibility for their actions, and the public's acceptance of direct access and direct reimbursement for services. The time has come for the initial professional education in physical therapy to culminate in the award of a doctorate in physical therapy or a doctor of science in physical therapy.

Compelling reasons that justify developing all professional education at that level include:

Demand. Physical therapists are aware of the constant demand for greater depth and breadth of knowledge in the structure and normal function of body systems and how body systems respond when function is disturbed by illness or trauma; skill in managing care to prevent movement dysfunction, to develop normal movement function throughout the life cycle, to maintain function as a natural process, and to restore movement function that has been impaired by illness or trauma; skill in communications and in the political process; skill in personnel and fiscal management; and skill in making ethical and clinical decisions.

Time. The time to complete current entry level baccalaureate and master's degree programs in physical therapy exceed that required for most other disciplines. The credit hours assigned for coursework in either kind of program usually is not a true representation of the actual hours spent in the classroom, laboratory, and treatment environments.

A well-designed professional doctorate would require three calendar years; the equivalent of the four academic years required to complete a professional degree in medicine, dentistry, or law.

Recruitment. As competition has grown for the available seats in existing programs, both the number and the quality of applicants has soared. That phenomenon can be expected to continue throughout the coming decades if the educational programs are challenging and the professional practice is rewarding personally and financially.

But the competition for able students will increase further as the pool of college-age applicants decrease. In the future, likely prospects for physical therapy must include those persons who are making career changes and some who have not been in the work force for several years. Doctoral study for entry into physical therapy will be appealing and satisfying to the highly qualified, older, committed candidate. The cost of education will not be viewed as a deterrent because graduates of doctoral programs can expect substantial incomes for their services and the cost of education can be recaptured in time.

Recognition. The practitioner who holds the title of *doctor* is accorded respect by the public, peers, and colleagues. To all, the doctoral degree represents years of intense and extensive study, suggests knowledge and competence in the field of study, and allows considerable freedom and independence in the practice of a chosen profession. In addition to the knowledge and competence, the title of doctor implies that the individual is ethical in practice. The resistance to direct access and direct reimbursement for services will have no validity when the preparation of the physical therapist is equivalent in time and title to that of "doctors" who currently control access to physical therapy services.

Opportunity. The depth and breadth of knowledge and skill acquired in a doctoral program will equip the clinician to function with independence; to identify problems that must be referred to another health care professional; to practice in less populated and remote areas of this and other countries; to serve as faculty members in educational programs; and to participate in research.

Other important reasons could be cited for establishing doctoral programs that focus on the preparation of a clinician generalist. One is the opportunity for practicing clinicians to return and earn a doctoral degree that may be more suited to their needs than a doctor of philosophy degree. Because the qualified practitioner could be expected to complete requirements for the doctoral degree in a shorter period than other candidates, a pool of experienced faculty members could be developed quickly.

The issue of clinical education continues to concern and perplex educational planners. Placing the initial professional preparation at the doctoral level would eliminate that concern. No amount of clinical education prior to completion of an education program will be considered enough. No one assumes that the newly graduated medical doctor is a finished product. Rather, the new physician is expected to complete a residency that may vary from two to seven years.

The new graduate from a doctoral program in physical therapy could be expected to spend an appointed time in a selected practice environment. That period of time could be designated as a postdoctoral fellowship, which implies continued learning and opportunity for growth under the tutelage of a preceptor or mentor. The standards applied to the period should be uniform, such as length of time, opportunities provided, and control. Matters such as salary, benefits, selection of preceptors and fellows, should be the prerogative of the participating practice environment. Removing concern for extended clinical experience from the academic faculty would leave them free to concentrate on other matters of substance.

Foundation for Professional Education

Entry-level education in physical therapy is meant to prepare a clinician generalist for practice. In any educational institution, the breadth and depth of the preparation provided are dependent on the available human, fiscal, and physical resources. The quality and quantity of those resources are related directly to the philosophy of the institution.

Each institution that offers an educational program in physical therapy has independent control of the requirements for admission to the program. Wide differences in the foundation required for professional education may contribute to variations in the quality of educational programs and, consequently, in the quality of graduates.

The clinician generalist in physical therapy is expected to be competent in the diagnosis of movement dysfunction and in creating and carrying out a plan of care designed to eliminate, alleviate, or minimize the identified dysfunction. In addition, the physical therapist is expected to communicate with individuals who have different educational, cultural, social, and economic backgrounds; act as an advocate for a patient or client and the family; participate in the political process at local, state, and national levels; market services; participate in research; teach patients, families, colleagues, and students; deal with third party payers for reimbursement of services; be a continuing learner; and be active in professional organizations.

Those expectations suggest that the foundation on which to build professional education must include the biological, physical, social, behavioral, and political sciences, mathematics, statistics, literature, history, philosophy, ethics, foreign languages, and communication skills.

The achievement of full professional status has eluded physical therapy. Because the public is the body that must perceive and acknowledge that an occupation embodies those characteristics common to a profession, considerable emphasis has been placed on clarifying and enhancing the image of physical therapy.

History shows us that the struggle could have been avoided. In a documented conversation with Sussman, Goode, a sociologist said:

> some professions come into existence when specialization occurs in a field or, as in the case of medicine, when more than one approach is used to the problems of illness. Medicine, purposely or by neglect, absolved its claim and consequently dentistry and social work emerged as professions with autonomy and legitimized power.[30]

According to Light,[31] however, physical therapy developed neither by absolution of a claim by medicine nor by neglect. Rather, physical therapy came into being because of the express needs of persons who suffered movement dysfunction from trauma or illness.

Instead of assuming autonomy and legitimized power, some of the early leaders insisted on maintaining an artificial and paternalistic relationship with physicians. Development in the shadow of medicine has given physical therapy a blurred image. To sharpen that image the following are recommended:

- Establish the *Doctor of Physical Therapy* degree (DPT) or the *Doctor of Science in Physical Therapy* (DScPT) for the initial professional preparation in physical therapy.
- Establishing an applied doctoral degree for practice

announces that physical therapy is a solemn undertaking that requires depth in knowledge and skill to practice. Further, physical therapy imposes obligations, responsibilities, and rights comparable to those assumed in medicine, law, and other such professions.

• Allow practicing physical therapists the opportunity to complete requirements for the applied doctorate in physical therapy. That opportunity should not be continued beyond a specified date after the doctoral degree is initiated.

• Eliminate educational programs that have not developed strong programs of research and have no plans to do so.

A profession thrives and continues to be useful to the public as new knowledge is uncovered and given practical expression in treatment procedures, equipment, and delivery of services. In 1967, Soffen reminded the profession of social work that.." the nature of education for a profession is such that it must be responsive to changing demands from the 'front lines' and at the same time give impetus to changing the field itself."[32]

Physical therapy educators cannot be allowed to ignore the fundamental obligation of the profession to change itself through research.

• Consolidate programs within a city, state, or region. Pool fiscal and faculty resources to create centers of excellence for learning, discovery of new knowledge, application of effective and efficient service, and introduction of new approaches to the management of care.

• Increase the size of entering classes annually to reflect a response to the need projected for the remaining years of the century. The need to add 3,800 new physical therapists each year to the 4,000 or more now being graduated annually means that the supply must be doubled. By increasing the class size to an average of 100 in 80 programs, the projected need could be met. Rather than open additional programs for 24 to 36 students, efforts should be directed toward maximum utilization of scarce resources, namely, faculty and funds, in developing larger programs.

• Organize all educational programs as separate schools within the university or as free-standing degree granting institutions in the community.

Existing programs within a geographic area could form a federation or a consortium to provide financial and other support to a single independent institution for physical therapy education. In one kind of arrangement, for example, participating institutions would continue to admit students and award the degree but the educational program would be administered apart form the several institutions.

• Establish a postdoctoral clinical fellowship program that allows the new graduate to select a general or a specialty program.

The postdoctoral fellowship program should be administered through a central agency that has responsibility for setting the standards of the program, accrediting the sites selected for participation in the program, and matching a candidate for the program with an approved site.

● Stagger enrollment throughout the year in a city, state, or region to allow treatment environments to have an even flow of students in clinical education, graduates in clinical fellowship programs, and potential candidates for first employment following completion of a fellowship program.

● Establish a central agency to process applications to all educational programs, administer a national admissions test, and collect and analyze data on applicants. By processing applications through a central agency, admission committees could have information in a standard format (designated by the individual institution); decisions by committees could be transmitted to candidates according to a plan; and the decisions of candidates could be made known without delay.

● Design educational programs that prepare clinicians to provide services in all parts of this nation, in developing nations, and in developed nations with a short supply of qualified physical therapists.

● Design programs to attract and retain minorities, persons making career changes, and older candidates who are making a career choice.

These recommendations are representative and not intended as an exhaustive list. The season for swift, decisive action in physical therapy education has come. Should the time pass unheeded, physical therapy may become, again, the handmaiden of others.

Summary

Our past has made us what we are today and our present will enable us to make us what we must become. Physical therapy of today has been shaped by the past. The future will have its roots in the present. Education is the foundation for that future.None of the issues presented in this chapter have simple or easy solutions. But none are without reasonable solutions that will benefit those we serve as well as all physical therapists.

References
1. Eccelesiastes 3:1(Old Testament)
2. Vogel E: The beginning of "modern physiotherapy." Phys Ther 56:15-21, 1976.
3. Department of Education: June 1986. American Physical Therapy Association, Alexandria, VA.
4. Hazenhyer IM: A history of the American Physiotherapy Association: Part 1. Prelude. Phys Ther Rev 26:3- 14, 1946.

5. American Women's Physical Therapeutic Association. Constitution: Article II. Objects. Phys Ther Rev 1:1-7, 1921.
6. Hazenhyer IM: A history of the American Physiotherapy Association: Part 2. Formative Years, 1926-1930, Phys Ther Rev 26:66-74, 1946.
7. Hazenhyer IM: A history of the American Physiotherapy Association: Part 3. The coming of age, 1931-1938. Phys Ther Rev 26:122-129, 1946.
8. Hislop HJ: The not-so-impossible dream. Phys Ther 55:1069-1080, 1975.
9. Verbatim Minutes: House of Delegates. Alexandria, VA, American Physical Therapy Association, June 1983.
10. Goode WJ: Encroachment, charlantanism and emerging professions: Psychology, sociology, and medicine. Am Soc Rev 25:902-1914, 1960. In: Sussman MB: Sociology and Rehabilitation. Washington, DC, US Department of Health, Education and Welfare, 1965.
11. Sussman MB: Sociology and Rehabilitation. Washington, DC, US Department of Health, Education and Welfare, 1965.
12. Educational Programs Leading to Professional Qualifications for the Physical Therapist, Approved/Accredited by the American Physical Therapy Association, 1928-1985. Alexandria, VA, American Physical Therapy Association, 1986.
13. Educational Programs Leading to Qualifications as a Physical Therapist. Phys Ther 67:1623-1626, 1987.
14. Verbatim Minutes: House of Delegates. Alexandria, VA, American Physical Therapy Association, June 1979.
15. Verbatim Minutes: House of Delegates. Alexandria, VA, American Physical Therapy Association, June 1979.
16. Hislop HJ, Worthingham CA: An analysis of physical therapy education and careers. Phys Ther Rev 35:228-241, 1955.
17. Gwyer JL: Attrition from physical therapy clinical practice. Unpublished doctoral dissertation; University of North Carolina, Chapel Hill, NC; 1983.
18. Blood H: Entry-level master's degree: A decade of experience. Phys Ther 64:208-212, 1984.
19. Morrison MA, Linder MT, Aubert EJ: Follow-up of graduates of one curriculum: 1956-1980. Phys Ther 62:1307-1312, 1982.
20. Johnson GR, Littell EH, Lehmkuhl D: Follow-up study of physical therapists completing a postbaccalaureate degree program between 1962-1971. Abstract. Phys Ther 67:790, 1987.
21. Hageman PA: Career profile of and feedback from graduates of a midwest curriculum. Phys Ther 68:79-84, August 1988.
22. Department of Practice: American Physical Therapy Association, Alexandria, VA.
23. 1987 Active Membership Profile Survey: Division of Research and Education. Alexandria, VA, American Physical Therapy Association, December 1987.
24. Department of Practice: American Physical Therapy Association, Alexandria, VA.

25. Johnsen O (ed): 1988 Almanac. New York, NY, Houghton Mifflin Co, 1987.

26. Report of the Task Force on Faculty Shortage in Physical Therapy. Alexandria, VA, American Physical Therapy Association, November 1985.

27. Accredited Bachelor's, Certificate, and Master's Degree Programs. Alexandria, VA, Department of Accreditation, American Physical Therapy Association, April 1988.

28. Nieland V: Personal Communication: August 1987. Department of Accreditation, American Physical Therapy Association, Alexandria, VA.

29. Occupational Outlook of Physical Therapy. Department of Practice. American Physical Therapy Association. (April) 1988 Spring.

30. Good WJ: Comment. In: Sussman MB: Sociology and Rehabilitation. Washington, DC, Department of Health, Education and Welfare, 1965.

31. Light I: Development and growth of new allied health fields. JAMA 210:114-120, 1969.

32. Soffen J: The school of social work and the profession. In: Faculty Development in Professional Education. New York, NY, Council on Social Work Education, 1967.

CHAPTER 2

Direct Access

Ernest Burch, Jr., BS, PT

The words used in the title of this chapter, direct access, refer to the ability of a consumer, the patient, to enter the health care system by going directly to the physical therapist who is to dispense their care. In this situation, a referral of the patient to a practitioner from the traditional source ie, the licensed medical doctor, dentist, or podiatrist is not required. This mode of practice has been referred to in the past as Independent Practice, Practice Without Referral, or Practice Independent of Practitioner Referrals.

The problems these three terms have presented historically for the physical therapy community are eliminated simply by the use of the term direct access. In discussions concerning independent practice, for example, individuals frequently posed the question of whether the speaker was referring to a free standing independent private practice or the ability to practice where a referral was not required. The use of the term direct access should ameliorate this problem. The use in the physical therapy community of the wording "practice without referral" has created and continues to create unneeded baggage in the form of antagonism from the medical community at large. Practice without referral connotes practice totally without need for or regard for referral, that is, a practice no longer related to the health care community. Nothing could be farther from the truth. The potential for improved relationships between physicians, our traditional colleagues, and physical therapists can be enhanced when physical therapists have the ability to practice offers direct access. Under direct access, therapists can be a valuable portal of entry into the health care system, and referrals can emanate than from physical therapists to other licensed health care practitioners. The words 'practice independent of practitioner referral' again brings the undesirable image that the therapist is practicing in a state of isolation from the rest of the health care world. In a jurisdiction where direct access is legal, direct access serves as a complement to the referral system and certainly is not a total replacement for the established custom.

Direct Access and Licensure

In reality, direct access does *not* mean *not* accepting referrals from physicians. In addition, it does *not* mean leaving the established medical community. However, it *does* mean a better understanding of roles; more responsibility for the therapist; better communication among all parties; and better patient care, which is of utmost importance. Better patient care and more cost-effective care should be the ultimate goal of direct access.

Whereas licensure has followed an evolutionary process that was based primarily on steps or acceptance within the legislative community, direct access has been more of a response to societal demands and the needs of the professionals involved. This latter phase is one of professional maturation. Although for physical therapy the acceptance of direct access has come more rapidly than licensure, at the time of this publication direct access still has not become legally acceptable in all states.

To illustrate the development of licensure for physical therapists as compared to Direct Access one can briefly review the history of these two professional milestones. The initial independent state licensure legislation for physical therapists was enacted by the New York legislature in 1926. Thirteen years later in 1939 regulations in Arizona required licensure of physical therapists. In 1941 Connecticut and Hawaii passed licensure legislation and in 1947 Maryland became the fifth state to require licensure. In the span of ten years, 1949-1959, twenty-eight additional states imposed mandatory as opposed to optional licensure laws. In 1971 legislators in Texas passed the law that mandated licensure in order to practice physical therapy. This law became effective in 1972. Forty-six years from start to finish were to pass before the licensure process was completed.

For comparison, by an act of legislature in 1979, Maryland became the first state to remove the requirement necessitating practitioner referral prior to treatment by a physical therapist. The citizens of that state thus were given direct access to licensed physical therapists. In the four years to follow, Arizona became the fifth state; within the next four years, sixteen more states passed legislation permitting direct access to physical therapy services. Therefore, while it took thirteen years to progress to where the second state required mandatory licensure to practice physical therapy and ten years have not yet elapsed from the enactment of the initial direct access legislation to where there are twenty-one state legislatures that have approved of this action. An additional nineteen state legislatures have now approved of evaluation without referral.

Development of Direct Access

Acceptance of the concept of direct access by physical therapists professional organization, the American Physical Therapy Association came after several false starts and was marked by episodes of significant misunderstanding among physical therapists themselves.

In 1973, a motion was introduced to the APTA House of Delegates by a member of the Board of Directors, Ms. Jane Mathews. That motion, RC 17-73, was passed by the House and essentially had the intent of Association endorsement of the principle of initial evaluation without practitioner referral. The motion also required that certain guidelines be developed by the Board of Directors. The guidelines were to stipulate the professional and ethical implications and the responsibilities of the physical therapists who would be engaging in evaluation without referral. Additionally, these guidelines were to be presented to the 1974 House of Delegates for consideration.

Confusion and opposition existed to a significant extent in the physical therapy community at that time. As a result, in 1976 the House passed a motion, RC 4-76, that rescinded the House action taken on RC 17-73 in 1973. Although this action reversed the decision made taken by the 1973 House, the support statement again reiterated the belief that the public needed and deserved an alternate route of entry into the traditional health care system. The statement also acknowledged that in light of the amount of confusion within the physical therapy community, there also must exist an even greater interpretation of problems in the health care system regarding the issue of direct access.

Between the years of 1976 and 1979, discussion of this topic continued to surface both in professional and informal arenas. In 1978, the House passed RC 42-78 that charged the Board of Directors to devise a plan for the development of physical therapy practice independent of practitioner referral. This plan was to be based on the identification of competencies that the therapist would be required to possess in order to practice in this manner. The body of the motion states that these were to include but not be limited to the following:

1. The physical therapy curriculum content necessary to achieve the identified competencies for practice independent of practitioner referral.
2. The revisions necessary to the *Standards for Accreditation of Physical Therapy Education Programs*.
3. A proposed time table for the accomplishment of curricula changes.
4. A draft of model legislative changes for state chapters.

Interim reports were to be presented to the House in 1979 and 1981, with a final report to the House scheduled for 1982. In 1979, however, two motions pertinent to this subject were passed by the House. The first, RC 18-79, independent practice, was introduced by the Maryland Chapter. This motion was designed to allow physical therapists to practice ethically in such jurisdictions where practice without practitioner referral currently was permitted legally. The support statement for that motion read as follows: "The Maryland Chapter offered this motion to help bring APTA Ethical Policies in line with the health care needs of the public as recognized in its statement of priorities (adopted by the House of Delegates in 1971 and reaffirmed in 1974). These priorities call for 'availability of health screening, preventive and early care, and timely referral for more extended care. . . ', and cannot be met unless the physical therapist is in a position to serve as first contact practitioner.

The change in policy is needed, also, to bring Association policies in line with current physical therapy practice in certain states and in the uniformed services."

It is interesting that the second paragraph of the support statement alludes to the fact that practice independent of practitioner referral already existed. That is, the legal recognition of direct access actually preceded the ethical recognition of this form of practice.

The motion was passed with a proviso that this policy not take effect until the following stipulations were met:

1. The *Standards for Physical Therapy Services* and the *Standards for the Physical Therapy Practitioner* are amended and approved by the House of Delegates to provide guidelines and minimal standards for practicing without practitioner referral.
2. The plan for development of physical therapy practice independent of practitioner referral (RC 42-78) is approved by the House of Delegates
3. The Board of Directors be charged to reassess its timetable for the completion of RC 42-78, giving the highest possible priority to completing this task by the 1980 House of Delegates.

The second pertinent motion passed in the 1979 House was RC 17-79, Initial Evaluation. This was introduced by the Board of Directors and stated in effect that it now was ethical for a physical therapist to provide evaluation and consultation without referral when it was permitted by state law. The support statement for this motion follows in its entirety. (It is interesting to note again a statement in the second paragraph that this practice already existed).

> The Board of Directors concurs with the Judicial Committee in:
> ● Recognizing that many persons in need of physical therapy services are not receiving same because they have not been processed through recognized referrals to physical therapists.
> ● Recognizing that assessment of potential patients is a necessary first step to entry into the treatment system.
> ● Believing that physical therapists have the professional qualifications to serve as an initial entry point for persons into the health care delivery system.

[Also] "various practice situations (now) exist in which medical referrals for initial entry into the health care system may not be necessary (eg, school systems). Ethical problems facing physical therapists working in these situations must be addressed.

Although the previous support statements indicate that practice without practitioner referral already existed, two motions debated in the 1980 House revealed that a degree of uncertainty was still present regarding referral relationships.

The support statement of a different motion, RC-81, introduced by the Missouri Chapter and presented to the 1981 House on referral relationships clearly establishes the basis for such a relationship. The motion in part states "that in a jurisdiction in which it is legally permissible a physical therapist ethically may treat patients within the limits of his/her knowledge, experience, and expertise without practitioner referral." The support statement is as follows:

The purpose of establishing criteria or guidelines for physical therapy practice without practitioner referral is to protect the patient. The mere inclusion of the requirement for a diagnosis does not accomplish this purpose and, in fact, places restrictions on the provision of services which far exceed those that currently exist under the referral requirement. A more valid method of protecting the patient is to establish criteria which address the primary issue of defining the role, responsibility and competence of the individual physical therapist.

In an action of equal importance in 1981, the Missouri Chapter also introduced the motion that finally stated clearly the philosophical position of the APTA that the physical therapist may be the entry point into the health care system and that this be a long term goal of the APTA. The adoption of this clear and concise philosophical statement now can serve as a guideline for actions concerning direct access that are necessary for future practice.

The actual goals and objectives for achieving physical therapy practice independent of practitioner referral were detailed in RC 88-82. This bill was introduced by the Board and passed by the 1982 House. This action assured the membership that the implementation of the policies would be attained by the professional organization.

Recognizing of the majority voice of the membership, the APTA took action on direct access that paralleled action take by chapters providing vigorous leadership in direct access legislation. The APTA actively supported the achievement of direct access legislation in all states and Commonwealths.

States began to pass legislation permitting direct access within their jurisdictions. Although the APTA had taken a stand on the issue, the legal conflicts in all states were far from being eliminated. Maryland was the first state to achieve direct access by the removal of the referral requirement. The history of the activities undertaken by the Maryland Chapter are of interest for several reasons. The Maryland Chapter can serve as a model for others. The Maryland Chapter took positive steps to establish direct access while the House of Delegates, APTA, debated the issue.

Direct Access History of Maryland

As in all professional organizations, there are times in the orderly process of planned changes in which unexpected events occur. Sometimes these unexpected events block the process of orderly change, but at other times, these unexpected events actually hasten the changes. The Association's long range plans to implement an orderly process to obtain direct access for physical therapists into the health care system were disrupted as some chapters moved in their own legislature arenas ahead of the Association's scenario of scheduled events. Carefully designed policies and guidelines of the Association were not being acted on as planned.

Each state had its own reasons for its timing of legislative action. Maryland's rationale essentially was to "strike while the iron was hot." In 1978 in Maryland, for example, occupational therapists obtained initial licensure and simultaneously received their licensure without referral. This was done with the understanding that sponsors of the Occupational Therapy Bill would assist the physical therapists in securing licensure without referral in the following year. In light of this providential opportunity, it seemed foolhardy for the physical therapists not to move as quickly as possible. Furthermore, because the occupational therapists had the privilege of treating in schools without waiting for referrals, the physical therapist's major goal was to seek these same rights.

Although the statutes that governed the practice of physical therapy at that time required verbal or written referrals, it was indeed fortunate that the law did not require a diagnosis or prescription for treatment to be given. This was not mandated because most orders for physical therapy did not include either a diagnosis or a prescription. This was a well-documented fact for the legislators during the legislative hearings on direct access in Maryland.

It was relatively easy to document that orders most frequently obtained the words "evaluate and treat," "PT," or simply "as necessary." Although the physical therapists had referrals to authorize treatments, they seldom had a prescription for care or a diagnosis of the patient's condition Frequently, some of those referrals that did prescribe treatment were not appropriate.

The physician-therapist relationship that existed at that time was built on an understanding and confidence in the level of expertise that each practitioner brought into the relationship. The mutual desire to ensure that the quality of care for the patient required that this confidence in the others abilities be justified. Physicians who gave orders to therapists that simply stated "back," or "shoulders," "PT" or even "evaluate and treat as needed" in effect were demonstrating this confidence in therapists to use their sound judgment in planning and in implementating the physical therapy regimen for those patients. Physical therapists also believed and had confidence that if they called physicians to advise them regarding such matters as the planned program, the inappropriatness of physical therapy in a particular instance, or the need for the physician to re-evaluate the patient in light of the therapist's findings, that the call would be accepted in good faith and would receive action. Confidence and judgment should be a two way street, and it usually was for the physician and the physical therapist. Direct access has enhanced this mutual confidence where it previously had existed and established it more firmly.

In 1979, primarily as a result of the passage of Public Law 94-142 that mandated that services such as physical therapy must be provided as needed within the educational programming of the handicapped child, an amendment to the Physical Therapy Practice Act was introduced in the Maryland legislature by the chairman of the House Environmental Affairs Committee. That amendment removed the discriminatory requirement that physical therapists practice only upon referral. This requirement was considered discriminatory because physical therapy was the only health profession restricted by law to physician referral. None of the more recently licensed professionals were similarly restricted (ie occupational therapists, speech therapists, nurses, psychologists, audiologists, or social workers).

Educators in the public school system were extremely frustrated when they found that they needed a referral to utilize a physical therapist in the school setting because they frequently could not get a physician to come into the school system to give such a referral. Consequently, they often decided to employ occupational therapists instead of physical therapists. That eliminated the need to fight for referrals or to track a physician down to make a referral for a student needing therapy.

Several physicians proposed that this referral problem could be eliminated by the use of blanket referrals. In fact, these blanket referrals still are used commonly in some nursing homes and extended-care facilities. What is the validity of a blanket referral? What is so sacred about a referral that simply states "evaluate every patient admitted?" What is the value in perpetuating the requirement that physical therapists must have a referral to evaluate or treat patients, no matter how vague the referral? Once the physician orders the evaluation, the physical therapist becomes his or her agent. The physician, however, is still responsible if any problems arise. Is it not more rational and effective that the physical therapist perform the evaluation; make an appropriate plan of care, if indicated, and then consult with the physician regarding the plan? In this manner, the onus of responsibility is shifted from the physician, where it most clearly exists with the blanket referral, to a more properly shared responsibility between the physician and the therapist.

Testimony to the Senate Economic Affairs Committee, quoted below, requesting support for HB 346 substantiates the referral problem and proposed legislative solutions. This bill passed three readings in the House without a single dissenting vote. Testimony included the following:

"The confidence of the medical profession in the physical therapists is reflected in present day referrals which usually read "physical therapy evaluation and treatment as indicated" or simply "physical therapy." Our profession has demonstrated its ability to practice in a competent and ethical manner, recognizing its own limitations. Safeguards, other than physician referral, already exist in our *Law and Regulations.*

Interestingly, other than the Medical Board, the Physical Therapy Board is the only health-related board to have promulgated a code of ethics. Effective treatment programs are based on a concept of reciprocal referral within the medical or educational model, with a mutual respect for the limitations and expertise of each member. As in the past, therapists' expertise (rather than the fact that a patient has been referred by a physician) will continue to assure safe quality of care."

The bill passed in the Senate Economic Affairs Committee unanimously. Thus, with only a single dissenting vote on the third reading in the Senate, the bill was forwarded to the governor for his signature and became law on July 1, 1979. Maryland thus became the first state to permit direct assess to physical therapy, by removal of the referral requirement.

Concerns about Effects of Direct Areas

Members of both the professional and lay population have expressed concerns regarding the effects of the passage of this type of legislation.

Specifically, they are concerned with its impact on the physical therapy profession and on the quality of care that will be dispensed. Examples of these legitimate concerns are:

- What will happen to malpractice insurance rates and who will protect the patient-consumer of physical therapy services?
- How physicians in general feel about direct access to physical therapy.
- How much more physical therapy is being given as a result of direct access legislation and what the cost will be to society.

Responses to these concerns can be formulated based on the actual experiences in states in which direct access has been legislated to date. What happened to malpractice insurance rates in these states? Did they escalate dramatically? The malpractice issue always is the source of considerable attention with some justification. In our present litigation-conscious society, the proliferation of the number of cases and the marked increase in the cost of settlements receives significant media attention. Society is much more "malpractice aware" than it was even ten or fifteen years ago. Malpractice insurance rates are based on the insurance carrier's experience with the actual occurrence of claims and the cost of the settlement of these claims. This experience factor is the basis for establishing rates for the practitioner in any given specialty. Hence, in medicine the higher premiums are in obstetrics, gynecology, orthopedics, and neurosurgery.

A letter dated February 20, 1987, written to the Honorable Chet Brooks, Chairman of the Senate Committee on Health and Human Services of the Texas Senate by Mr. Donald F. Lang, President of Maginnis and Associates, Professional Insurance Administrators, follows:

RE: Practice Without Referral

Dear Senator Brooks:

We understand your Committee is considering a piece of Legislation that would allow the physical therapist to practice without referral; namely Senate Bill No. 170.

Our firm as a Major Administrator of Professional Liability Insurance for Physical Therapists has been monitoring claims in those jurisdictions where practice without referral is allowed: Specifically, Alaska, Arizona, California, Kentucky, Maryland, Massachusetts, Nebraska, Nevada, North Carolina, South Dakota, Utah and West Virginia. It is my understanding that California and Nebraska are jurisdictions in which the therapist has been able to practice without referral for a considerable period of time. As of this writing, we have no firm evidence that practice without referral has had a negative impact on professional liability.

It would be normal, from an underwriter's approach to expect that when the therapist is practicing independent of the physician, claim experience might be less favorable than that where a physician is involved. Again, we do not find this to be the case at the present time. I can only suggest to you that the professional therapist utilizes every viable tool available in order to provide the patient with the best care possible. I would also suggest that in those areas where practice without referral has been allowed, the truth of the matter is that the therapist counsels with the physician in cases where there would be any questions whatever as to what might be proper in the handling of that patient. The less professional therapist is going to be more subject to losses with or without the restriction of requiring physician referral.

The number of incidents in the entire physical therapy area has been steadily increasing, as have been the dollar values of judgments in malpractice actions. These two factors in addition to others have had a negative effect on the pricing of professional liability coverage for physical therapists, but again that effect seems to be across-the-board and not a function of practicing with or without a referral. It is our intent to continue to monitor our therapy program.

Sincerely,
Donald F. Lang

The second concern regarding the safety of the patient-consumer also is addressed in the letter quoted above. In addition, states that allow direct access to physical therapy still maintain the State Laws and Regulatory Boards that govern the practice of physical therapy, (in the same manner as before passage of the direct access legislature.)

How do physicians, in general, think about the question of direct access? Although the medical community is divided as to the reaction to the passage of independent practice, a significant number of physicians think that it was "about time". Because physical therapists know more about physical therapy by education and experience than medical practitioners, they are more qualified to evaluate and initiate physical therapy. In addition, direct access removed the responsibility of referral from many physicians who were reluctant to assume that responsibility. That is, the referral reading as "PT" or "evaluate and treat as necessary" actually was a mandate from the physician to the physical therapist to practice physical therapy. Prior to direct access legislation many physicians who used these broad referrals for physical therapy actually abdicated the responsibility to evaluate the patient for treatment by a physical therapist.

Concerns about over-utilization of physical therapy and fears about increased costs can be put to rest by statistics from the health insurance industry. Blue Cross and Blue Shield currently pay for physical therapy procedures without a physician's signature in some states that have direct access. It seems unlikely that all this would not have occurred if their statistics indicated that direct access drastically increased costs. The insurance industry, as well as society, is interested in cost containment. Direct access to physical therapy actually can reduce costs to the consumer by eliminating a physician visit in which a physician simply writes a blanket referral.

Let us look at one last objection to independent practice. Patients may be placed at greater risk because physical therapists are not qualified to determine what actually is wrong with patients. The following hypothetical scenario effectively analyzes this argument:

A 50-year-old gentleman is in search of care for low back pain. His symptoms could have their origin in any one of several problems: musculoskeletal dysfunction, postural abnormality, kidney disease, spinal cord tumor, aortic aneurysm, protruding or herniated intervertebral disk, degenerative joint changes, spondylitis, spondylolisthesis, or even emotional stress. This list of possible problems is not exhaustive, but will suffice for the purpose of this argument. The patient has several courses of action to seek care for his low back pain.

Option 1

He can take anyone of the over-the-counter advertised pain relievers for "X" days. If the pain reliever does not work to his satisfaction, he might use a heating pad and take one of the advertised "extra-strength pain relievers." This regimen may relieve his problem or it may simply mask the problem for a period of time and, thus, delay potentially effective treatment.

Option 2

The patient can go to his family practitioner who may prescribe some of the same measures used in the self-care Option 1. The family practitioner, during an initial visit, would not most likely refer the patient for any diagnostic tests but would simply perform a routine examination to rule out problems that are not of musculoskeletal origin. If symptoms persist or increase, however, the family practitioner would conduct further testing or refer the patient to a specialist.

Option 3

The patient could go to a licensed physical therapist who would, within the limits of his or her expertise, assess the patient's complaints. He or she would obtain a subjective and clinical history and assess posture, muscle function, joint function, and nervous system integrity. The physical therapist, if appropriate, then would plan and administer a therapeutic program. As time progressed, the physical therapist would monitor the patient's response to the treatment. If the response to the treatment regimen was not positive, or if other complaints or signs emerged, the physical therapist would make a referral to an appropriate medical practitioner. Similar referral also could be made at the initial evaluation if symptoms and examination findings indicated that physical therapy was inappropriate or contraindicated in this case.

Option 4

The individual could go to a licensed health practitioner other than a medical practitioner or physical therapist. Without describing what might be done in this situation or speculating the outcome, one thing seems certain; if symptoms were to persist or increase in this situation, it is less likely that he would be referred to an appropriate medical practitioner as he would in Option 3.

Option 5

In the worst case scenario, he could go to any one of the several kinds of unlicensed, self-proclaimed health practitioners and thus delay or eliminate care by an educated and state regulated health care practitioner.

Which of the above options poses the greater risk to the gentleman if, in fact, his problem is not of musculoskeletal origin but one of the potentially life-threatening problems? One could argue that, except for Option 2, Option 3 is a more legitimate and safer choice for this individual to enter the health care system and reach appropriate care for his low back pain. The physical therapist is trained to assess the pain from a neuro-musculoskeletal perspective and therefore is more likely to identify if the pain is not consistent with the usual neuro-musculoskeletal symptoms. If that were the case, the physical therapist would make an appropriate referral. The same cannot be said with confidence for the other options listed.

Plans for the Future

Common sense and the ever present threat of malpractice liability have governed practice effectively under direct access legislation. Societal constraints will continue to operate; that is, the state regulatory boards will continue to insure that the physical therapist practices within the rules and regulations promulgated by these governmental boards. The regulations are for the protection of the consumer, and the legal restrictions exist in the absence as well as the presence of direct access legislation. In jurisdictions where direct access is legal, it is not mandatory; therefore, the physical therapist who wishes to practice in the traditional referral-based type of situation may continue to do so. Direct access and referral-based practice can and do co-exist.

The APTA has an ongoing commitment to assist the state and commonwealth components, which do not currently have direct access, in their efforts to obtain the passage of this enabling legislation. These efforts consist of advice and guidance.

Additionally, some resources are being developed such as brochures and audiovisual aids. These are being developed to drive home the assertion that the academic and clinical accomplishments of physical therapists lead to the irrefutable conclusion that physical therapists, in fact, are qualified and prepared to provide a cost-effective entry point for patients into the traditional health care system.

CHAPTER 3

Referral for Profit

Philip Paul Tygiel, BS, PT

"Referral for profit arrangements involving physicians and physical therapists are like a cancer eating away at the ethical, moral and financial fiber of our profession."[1]

Attributed to Charles M. Magistro, PT
past APTA President
22nd Mary McMillan Lecture.

In June of 1979, after several years of discussion, investigation, and debate, the American Physical Therapy Association's House of Delegates passed a motion calling on its Board of Directors to devise a plan to assist chapters in making legislative changes that would preclude physical therapists from practicing in arrangements in which referring practitioners could profit as a result of referring patients for physical therapy. Then and since then, no other single issue has been the subject of as much debate, scrutiny, understanding, and misunderstanding.

The position was challenged frequently in the ensuing years, but the House always remained firm in its resolve that referral for profit is not acceptable.

Resolution to Oppose Referral For Profit

In 1981, the following resolution, which broadened the Association's approach to the problem of referral for profit, was passed:

Whereas, The APTA is committed to meet the physical therapy needs of the people and advocates a system of delivery which results in the most economical and highest quality of patient care;

Whereas, When physicians can profit as a result of referring patients for physical therapy, conflicts have arisen in the delivery of physical therapy which influence both the cost and quality of these services and which also interfere with the consumer's choice of physical therapist;

Whereas, It may not be in the best interest of the consumer for the physical therapist to practice directly or indirectly under arrangement with a referring physician or group of physicians who, as a result of referring patients to the physical therapist, derive personal income as a direct or indirect result of the referral;

Whereas, Spokesmen in medicine have openly voiced concerns about physicians deriving income from health care except those fees earned from their own services;

Whereas, The APTA's House of Delegates has provided direction to assist chapters in amending physical therapy practice acts to preclude physical therapists from having, or entering into, arrangements with health care practitioners where such arrangements in any manner result in an unearned income for the referring practitioner;

Whereas, The Judicial Committee of the APTA recognizes the ethical problems posed in such situations but also recognizes that federal anti-trust provisions prevent a professional association from outrightly prohibiting any type of employment relationship; now, therefore, be it

Resolved, That the Board of Directors initiate a program that will educate physical therapists about problems that arise in referral for profit situations.

Resolved, To open dialogue with appropriate organizations, including the American Hospital Association and the American Medical Association and its specialty boards, about the possible unethical practice in physicians owning physical therapy practices.

Resolved, That the chapters be encouraged to seek legislative alternatives to resolve the problems inherent in such arrangements as set forth above.

It should be understood that this resolution was not aimed solely at physical therapists who were employed by physicians in physician-owned physical therapy services (POPTS) but also aimed at physical therapists who worked in hospital situations in which physicians received a percentage of the department's income in return for referring patients, and at physical therapists who worked in private settings and paid fees back to referring physicians to get their referrals. The resolution did not apply to physical therapists who worked in physician's offices and rented space at a reasonable flat rate, however. In those situations the physician profited only as a landlord and could not increase income by referring more patients for therapy.

Task Force Delineates Problems

In response to the resolution, a task force was formed by the APTA Board in early 1982. Its recommendations were approved by the Board at their March, 1982 meeting. The report included the following problem statement:

In referring patients to physical therapists, referring practitioners may require that they receive direct or indirect financial rewards for making the referral. Such a practice can obviously lead to patient exploitation, an abuse the APTA must oppose.

Since the referring practitioner is held in a position of trust by the patients served, patients normally place unquestioning reliance on the physician's judgment. Patients are not usually in a position to identify overuse or misuse of the referred services. When a physician can gain financially from the referral process, the potential for violation of the patient's trust is increased. The APTA believes a significant number of such situations exist. The Association further believes these practices harm the public, the medical profession, and the physical therapy profession.

Specific areas of potential patient abuse are:

Patients may be referred when services are not actually needed.

Patients may be referred for more services (type, quantity) than are actually needed.

Patients may not have made available to them the physical therapy expertise best suited to their needs.

Patient's freedom of choice in selecting a physical therapist is limited.

Policy Statement 1983

In 1983, the APTA House drafted the following statement, which was amended and made stronger in 1985.(The amendments are in italics.)

The American Physical Therapy Association is opposed to situations in which physical therapists or physical therapist assistants are employed by or under agreement with referring practitioners or organizations owned by referring practitioners and in which the referring practitioner receives compensation either directly or indirectly as a result of referring for, prescribing, or recommending physical therapy. *No referring practitioner should bill or be paid for a service which he does not perform; mere referral does not constitute a professional service for which a professional charge should be made or for which a fee may be ethically paid or received.* The Association believes that these arrangements offer a serious potential for abuse in the provision of physical therapy. The Association further believes that the effective provision of physical therapy will be enhanced if such arrangements are avoided.

Interestingly, the words in the amended portion were taken directly from the American Medical Association's 1981 Judicial Committee Opinions.

Current Trends

As recently as 1987, some individuals have challenged the House's firm stance on this issue, but once again the House's original position clearly was upheld.

A frequently asked question is, "Why has this issue become so important?" Years ago, it was considered better to have a physical therapist working for a physician than to have an untrained aide performing physical therapy in the doctor's office. At one time, it was even considered honorable to work for a physician; a great opportunity. In fact, the idea of physical therapists working privately and not under the direct on-site supervision of doctors was frowned upon.

Times, medicine, and physical therapy have all changed considerably since then. When "then" was, however, is not really clear because the transition was a metamorphosis that varied in time and place. Nonetheless, most physicians could then, if they had to, perform the same skills that physical therapists performed. Physicians did not perform physical therapy, however, because of time limitations and because in doing so they would have increased health care costs. They therefore hired physical therapists to perform these tasks. Additionally, physical therapists in most cases lacked the ability to work independently.

Today, however, the combination of knowledge and skills used by physical therapists is not in the realm of physicians. The knowledge and skills are unique to the physical therapy profession and, therefore, it is up to physical therapists to take professional responsibility for their administration.

This professional responsibility is the keystone of the opposition to referral for profit. The position is designed not to protect physical therapists from being exploited but to protect the public from being abused solely for financial gain.

Public Trust

Now, it certainly is true that the potential for patient abuse through overuse or misuse of services exists in all professional situations. In fact, that is the nature of professions. "Because of the importance of the professional functions and the inability of the receiver of these functions to assess the quality of service, a relationship of trust must exist between the professional and the patient. When the physician recommends surgery, the patient (having little ability to validate the professional's conclusion) must trust that this recommendation is made in the best interest of the patient, and not made merely to provide monetary gain to the physician providing the service.[2] The professional dictates what is good or evil for clients who have no choice but to accede to professional judgment. Here, the premise is that because clients lack the requisite theoretical background, they cannot diagnose their own needs or discriminate among the range of possibilities for meeting them.[3] "The professions are concerned with matters that are vital to the health or well being of their patients. In practicing a profession, practitioners use highly specialized technical knowledge, which patients or clients do not possess. Because patients lack knowledge, opportunity exists for exploitation of patients by professionals. Because of the vital nature of professional services, the consequences to patients of such exploitation are severe. The smooth functioning of professions therefore requires that practitioners consider the needs of patients as having paramount importance, relegating the material needs of practitioners to an inferior position.[2]"

"One measure of social sanction is the granting of exclusive rights of practice through the licensing power of the state. Although such licensing attempts to protect the public from incompetent practitioners, it also frequently creates a relationship of trust between society and the professionals.

"The extent of this trust also is a measure of the degree of social sanction; however, it is measured by a lack of the exercise of sovereign power. Given the legal monopoly inherent in professional licensing, the failure of society to impose further controls on a profession, sanctions by implication, the performance of self-regulation of the profession."[2]

Additionally, because professionals enjoy relationships of trust with patients or clients, "the fiduciary relationship between professional and client involves certain restrictions on the professional man's method of charging. It requires that the practitioner shall be financially disinterested in the advice he gives or, at least, that the possibility of conflict between duty and self-interest shall be reduced to a minimum."[4]

Conflict of Interest

In all professional situations, potential conflicts of interest exist. Practitioners are supposed to recommend only services that are in the best interest of their patients. Many of these recommendations will also benefit practitioners by enhancing their incomes, but that enhancement should not be considered when practitioners determine what to recommend. These conflicts do exist, however, and provide temptations that, unfortunately, are not always resisted properly by professionals.

There are, however, two different categories of conflict of interest. "A distinction should be made between those conflicts which are inherent in the professional relationship and those which are voluntarily created by the practitioner. The former require restraint by the professional to insure that there is no patient exploitation. The latter, since they are an unnecessary part of the professional relationship, should be avoided."[2]

When a surgeon, for example, sees a patient with a potential surgical condition, he can recommend nonsurgical treatment or he can recommend surgery. He certainly can make more money by recommending the surgery. The patient must trust and hope that the surgeon will choose the course of treatment that is in the patient's best interest. This type of conflict is inherent in the surgical profession. There is no way it can be avoided.

In physical therapy, there are similar inherent conflicts. A therapist, for example, can derive an increase in income by using more modalities and seeing a patient more frequently. The patient must trust and hope that the therapist will choose only the treatment procedures and the frequency of treatment that will aid the patient most effectively.

Another example of unnecessary conflict of interest in the professional relationship is a physician's ownership of a pharmacy. In owning a pharmacy, a physician would be placed voluntarily in a position where income would be derived by prescribing drugs and having patients fill their prescriptions only at the physician's pharmacy. This conflict of interest can and should be avoided. The pharmacy profession declared this practice to be unethical and worked to make it illegal as well.

Voluntary ownership of physical therapy services by physicians similarly creates an unnecessary conflict of interest. "When the position of trust is regarded as extending to a profession as a whole, it is seen that certain common commercial practices are incompatible with the rendering of professional services; and from these practices the professional man is required to abstain."[4] Physicians who employ or profit from physical therapists receiving their referrals are, therefore, acting unprofessionally. Physical therapists should follow the lead of pharmacists and refuse to participate in the unprofessional conduct of others.

Several questions have been raised: Why prohibit profit for referral? Why not just address the problem of overutilization and misutilization of services in all settings? Why can't the APTA's Judicial Committee and the various state licensing boards handle these problems of patient abuse?

The Association's Judicial Committee and legal counsel have determined that their procedures as outlined are insufficient to handle the situation. The Judicial Committee has no subpoena power and only can censure therapists or suspend them from APTA membership. The committee cannot properly investigate overutilization or collusion, and it cannot, nor should it be able to, stop physical therapists from practicing. Curtailing practice remains under the jurisdiction of the states. For this reason, the Judicial Committee and legal counsel assisted in the drafting of the 1981 resolution and encouraged its passage.

State boards operating under most current practice acts also would have difficulty dealing with overutilization. The biggest problem would be the impossibility of proof and enforcement. Even a physician and a physical therapist, obviously working in collusion and gouging the public by overtreating, could defend themselves by stating that in their professional opinion the services were required. It is unlikely that they would be charged with collusion at all because unsuspecting patients lack the knowledge to judge that they have been taken advantage of.

Referral for Profit Examples

Following are examples of situations in which patient's rights obviously were abused because they saw a physician who profited as a result of referrals for physical therapy. No charges were filed against any of these physicians or physical therapists because of the previously stated reasons.

1. The patient was a stroke victim who had difficulty using his right hand. He saw an orthopedic surgeon for surgery on his hand. Physical therapy was needed for his rehabilitation. The physician had a therapist working for him who had no particular expertise in treating hands, just routine experience. The patient lived on the east side of the town; the orthopedic surgeon was some 20 miles away on the west side. The patient was required to drive across town to see the physician's physical therapist. Several excellent hand physical therapists were located much closer to the patient's home and could have served him just as well, if not better.

2. The patient was injured on the job and complained of left midback pain. She was seen by a physiatrist and her condition was diagnosed as myofibrositis. The patient was referred to his physical therapist. The patient did not like the physical therapist nor the selected treatment,

which was transcutaneous electrical nerve stimulation. She called the insurance company and told them this; they advised her to consult the physician again. She saw the physician one week later and told him she did not like the therapist or the treatment and would not like to go back to his physical therapist. The physician reexamined her at that visit and said he then found nothing wrong with her. He also said she had to go back to work and closed her case.

She was still in pain and sought consultation with another physician. He examined her, diagnosed her condition as a mechanical back problem, and referred her to physical therapy. The physical therapist she was referred to had training in the treatment of spinal conditions. The patient was evaluated,treated with mobilization, and the pain was eliminated. Unfortunately, the patient had to hire a lawyer to have the case reopened so that she could have her bills paid and so she would not lose money for taking time off from work.

3. A physical therapist was working in a physician's office and maintaining high ethical standards, despite the potential conflict of interest in working for three orthopedic surgeons. Two of the surgeons were partners in the firm and one was an employee. The physical therapist recognized his own limitations in certain areas. In situations in which he felt he lacked the skill or equipment to treat the patient properly, he requested that the patients be referred to other physical therapists in the community who had either more skill for treating the particular condition or the exercise equipment more suitable for ther problems. Interestingly, the orthopedic surgeon who was an employee regularly approved these requests. The two surgeons who were owners of the facility routinely denied these requests.

4. A physical therapist who works for an orthopedic surgeon is well-skilled in treating spinal conditions but has no particular expertise in treating hands. The orthopedic surgeon is involved in a good deal of hand surgery and requires his patients to see his physical therapist. In the area, there are at least four well-qualified hand therapists, either occupational therapists or physical therapists. Particular problems arise frequently in the area of splinting for these patients with hand problems. Splinting techniques require special skills; however, the physician's physical therapist does not have good training in those techniques. Very often, the patients have to be referred elsewhere for resplinting at an additional cost to the patients.

5. A patient was injured while working at a local hospital. She complained of a cervical pain syndrome. She had a previous medical history of a similar problem that was treated successfully by a local physical therapist. She was referred by the hospital emergency room to a physiatrist who has physical therapists working for him. He told her that she needed physical therapy and that she should see one of his therapists. The patient requested to see a different physical therapist, one that she had seen previously, but the physiatrist refused. He insisted that she see his physical therapists.

On the first visit the patient saw a physical therapist who did not work regularly in that office and had little training, if any, in spinal orthopedics. She had no relief and requested to see the physical therapist that she had seen previously. This request was refused. On the second visit, she saw a physical therapist in that office who did have training in spinal management and she did have some relief. On the third visit, she was sent to another office owned by the same physician and was treated by an aide. She had no relief and requested to see the physical therapist of her choice. Again, this was refused. On the fourth visit, she was seen by yet another physical therapist with no advanced training in this type of treatment. He provided no relief. She again requested to see the physical therapist of her choice and was refused. She finally went to another physician and was able to go to the physical therapist she wanted to see.

6. A group of physicians employs physical therapists. This particular group charges for treatment by the modality. The more modalities used on a patient, the more the patient is charged. One of the physical therapists found that when treating patients with low back syndrome who also had radicular pain down the leg, he received orders from the physicians not only for treatments such as diathermy, ice massage, massage, and exercise for the low back but for separate modalities such as ultrasound or electrical stimulation for radicular pain down their legs. The physical therapist believed that the additional treatment was unnecessary and resulted in an increased cost to the patient. He attempted to refuse these treatments and was told by the physicians to "play ball or get off the team".

The physical therapist not only got off the team, but he quit physical therapy and went to chiropractic school because he did not want to have to work under physicians again.

All of these situations would have been avoided had the physical therapist involved not entered into a <u>voluntary</u> conflict of interest in the first place.

Future Considerations

Physical therapists must do their best always to act ethically in their individual practices. Physical therapists and the APTA are guardians of the public's trust and, therefore, must do as much as possible to protect the public from abuses by anyone who is in or related to the profession. Therapists, therefore are professionally, morally, and ethically obligated to eliminate these voluntary conflicts of interest.

Some people speculated that the advent of direct access to physical therapy eventually would lead to the natural demise of referral for profit. This has not proven to be true. In fact, referral for profit settings seem to be on the rise. This rise may well be, in part, a direct result of the medical economic trend of the 1980s. The prospective payment system, the health maintenance organizations, and other types of prepaid plans all have cut into the physician's traditional income. Additionally, changes in tax laws have seriously reduced tax shelter opportunities. To counter this, many physicians began to look at alternate sources of income. Some discovered that ownership of physical therapy services and other businesses to which they referred could be quite a lucrative income source. These were businesses they could enter with minimal risk because they could control the patient flow.

Economic jargon of the 1980s has begun to creep into the referral-for-profit picture. Terms such as "joint venture" and "limited partnership" now are heard. In a cover letter describing one such venture to potential physician investors the opening paragraph reads as follows:

> As a colleague interested in protecting my own future, I have become involved in a very interesting project that may be a help in protecting your future also. In spite of having my own physical therapy unit for years, at least half of my patients have been referred to physical therapy facilities out of my control. I have also lost much potential income from these outside referrals. This is no longer necessary in my opinion.

The proposal goes on to tell doctors how they can increase their income by investing in a physical therapy office and how they can make more money referring more patients.

These ventures raised new questions to the Association members about referral for profit. In response, the APTA's House of Delegates approved the following definition of referral for profit at its 1986 meeting: "A referral for profit relationship is any situation in which referring practitioners receive compensation as a result of referrals."

Physical therapists must guide their profession's growth properly, being careful to keep the best interest of the public served as the foremost consideration. They must research and analyze all of the aspects of any given problem carefully. They must take the best from what other professions have done as they emerged and must avoid the mistakes that others have made already. In some cases, physical therapists can follow the lead of others; however, in other cases they must forge new roads. With regard to referral for profit, the physical therapy profession would do well to follow the lead of the pharmacy profession. Pharmacy has been described as "a highly specialized calling, which may rise to the dignity of a true profession or sink to the level of the lowest commercialism, according to the ideals, the ability, and the training of those who practice it."[5]

The same may be said of physical therapy. Which of the two roads physical therapy takes depends on physical therapists both individually as they choose to practice and collectively as they choose to behave as a profession.

References

1. Magistro CM: Physician-Physical Therapist Financial Arrangements. Read at Combined Section Meeting of the American Physical Therapy Association, San Diego, CA. February 14-17, 1982.
2. Myers J: Remington's Pharmaceutical Sciences. Easton, PA, Mack Publishing Company, 1970, pp 20-25.MC
3. Greenwood E: In Nosow S, Form WH, (eds): Man, Work and Society, New York, NY, Basic Books, 1962, pp 210-6.
4. Carr-Saunders AM, Wilson PA: The Professions. Oxford, England, The Clarendon Press, 1933, pp 426-432.
5. LaWall CH: Four Thousand Years of Pharmacy. Philadelphia, PA, Lippincott Co, 1920, pp v.

CHAPTER 4

Specialization in Physical Therapy

Colleen Kigin, MS, PT

In any line of endeavor it is very easy for one to drift into a daily routine . . . Many of us perhaps gradually lost the habit of real thinking, and unless there is a constant probing of incentive, we fall into this crime of routine which is unfair to ourselves, our patients, and our profession. Following the war, [WW I] the incentive was ever present. Every time we change our position and take on new responsibility it is present. But after we have made our contacts, feel our position secure, we are often apt to drift.[1]

The beginnings of the physical therapy profession in the United States stem from the inauguration of the Division of Special Hospital and Physical Reconstruction by the Surgeon General's office on August 22, 1917. With the development of the field of physical therapy, courses of study that ranged from four to six weeks duration just after World War I rapidly progressed to such programs as the one-year program at the New Haven School of Physiotherapy in 1925.[2] The director of the New Haven School commented that the faculty members found it as difficult to encompass the work in one year as they had found for the shorter course. The director went on to point out that the curriculum needed to include more anatomy, physiology, theory, and practice in all phases of physiotherapy. The additional option of one year postgraduate study was available by 1927.

Early in the profession, the quest for increasing skill in particular areas of physical therapy resulted in postgraduate courses such as those offered at New Haven or at the Harvard Medical School. A Harvard course offered in August 1927 was advertised in the Physiotherapy Review as a course designed for graduates of physical education, nursing, and physiotherapy specializing in orthopedics.[3]

These courses did not develop as a result of casual interest or basic review.

The clinicians of the 1920s found themselves challenged in areas of care that required special study and increased clinical skill.[4] Specialization, therefore, is not new to our profession; however, the development of the structure to formally recognize clinical specialists did not occur until the late 1970s, with the first certification in 1985.

The profession now has the responsibility to further investigate the impact of this process on ourselves, our patients, and the health care community. Now is not the time to feel secure and perhaps allow ourselves to drift. Complacency or feeling that we "have arrived" is no more tolerable in the present than it was when Emily Wellington spoke to her colleagues in 1927.

This chapter will provide a history of certifying clinical specialists in the United States, including a review of the process necessary to establish this certification process and of the present and potential future impact of specialty certification on the profession.

Development of the Certification Process

Recognition of the specialist has occurred through a number of back doors. This is due to many factors, but perhaps the most prevalent has been the concern of clinicians regarding the formal commitment to such a process. The profession has observed pioneers in various areas of physical therapy who carve a nitch in the broader concept of the profession. These outstanding clinicians often are known by rumor or reputation.[5] The treatment developed by these pioneers may be regarded suspiciously or embraced with little understanding of the physiologic rationale or appropriate indications for use. The recognition afforded these clinicians as well as the techniques they may have developed has been hesitant; the ability, then, to recognize other clinicians' skills in practicing particular techniques has been nonexistent and many times unwanted.[5]

In 1973, a few members of the American Physical Therapy Association decided that the time had come to present the concept of formal recognition of specialists to the membership. George Soper of the Iowa chapter brought the motion to the House of Delegates which read:

> I move that (1) it shall be the policy of the American Physical Therapy Association to identify and publicly recognize specialties within physical therapy; (2) the Board of Directors study the feasibility of and methods for establishing specialties in physical therapy and that the Board's findings be reported back to the 1975 House of Delegates.[6]

The rationale for this motion is perhaps more or as important to the profession as the motion. The rationale reads:

> A growing number of physical therapists are involved in specialization or concentration in certain areas such as electrodiagnosis, cardiopulmonary care, neurological care and musculoskeletal care. Some physical therapists are seeking and accepting certification in these areas in associations external to the American Physical Therapy Association.

Each of these areas of specialization represents bodies of knowledge that have long been identified as falling within the total purview of physical therapy. It is therefore entirely appropriate and fitting that the American Physical Therapy Association should give recognition for special qualification in these areas within its membership.[6]

The House decided to form a task force to evaluate the concept of specialization. The task force was composed of Nancy Watts, Ron Peyton, and Art Nelson. This task force in turn brought a report to the 1975 House, which resulted in the House passing a policy statement on the recognition of specialists in physical therapy.[7]

In the process of developing the policy statement, this task force gathered information on the nature of specialization in other fields. They also did a survey to determine how broad the interest of the membership of the APTA was in such a process. The results of the survey were as one might expect; very mixed, with respondees either opposed vehemently or very supportive of the process. The task force decided that what they would not want to do was foster fragmented boards developing outside the APTA and, even with mixed survey results, that the profession owed the practitioners credentials in speciality areas. However, the task force also heard the opposition and did not want to create a system that was divisive within the APTA (personal communication, N. Watts, October 1986).[8] They therefore proposed a process with the following assumptions, which were presented to the House in 1975:

1. Formal recognition . . . could benefit both physical therapists and the public by promoting high standards of practice, rewarding excellence in clinical practice, and facilitating referral of patients with special needs.

2. Recognition . . . will be most beneficial . . . designed to indicate excellence in performance rather than narrowness of interest.

3. A plan . . . must propose a practical method for evaluation of individual competency . . .

4. [The] development . . . will be costly . . . and cannot proceed until the nature of specialized and advanced general practice has been clearly defined.

5. Some active interest now exists for . . . certification, however, the April 1974 membership survey and February 1975 chapter responses . . . indicate that at the present only a very small fraction of Association membership actively support immediate action . . .

6. [The] APTA can act most constructively . . . through comprehensive long-range planning rather than by piecemeal responses . . . [7]

The Section on Orthopaedics was frustrated with this report, believing that the process essentially would be at a standstill (personal communication, S. Burkart, February 1987).[9] Therefore, a motion was brought before the same House by Iowa to establish a second task force to look into the process further.[8] This second task force was to involve sections of the APTA that expressed an interest in such a process. This motion passed, and a second task force was appointed for further development of the process.

The policy statement proposed by the initial task force and passed by the 1975 House has formed the very basis of the process. The original criteria for development included the following:

The process will be 1) voluntary, 2) unrestrictive, 3) coordinated, 4) financially independent, 5) responsive to public interest, 6) based on existing

```
┌─────────────────────────────────────────────┐
│              FIGURE 4-1                       │
│        Task Force Members—1975                │
│                                               │
│           Robert Bartlett, Chair              │
│              Pamela Catlin                    │
│              Carol Erickson                   │
│              Carolyn Heriza                   │
│               Jack Hofkosh                    │
│                Scot Irwin                     │
│              Ann McColley                      │
│              Roger Nelson                      │
│              Stanley Paris                     │
│              Ronald Peyton                     │
│             Dorothy Pinkston                   │
│              Jeanne Schenck                    │
│              George Soper                      │
│             Nancy Thompson                     │
└─────────────────────────────────────────────┘
```

patterns of practice, and 7) designed to restore the growth of clinical theory and practice.[7]

The only criteria that is not currently fulfilled is number 4, financial independence. The goal of financial independence is discussed later in this chapter.

The second task force was to do the following:

1. Identify and define areas of specialization.
2. Explore needs for methods of establishing a certification system.
3. Define the structure and function of the certification body.[8]

The task force was comprised of the representatives from each section wishing to participate and the appointees selected by the Board of Directors (Fig.4-1). This task force met for three years and developed the guidelines for recognition of clinical specialization, including the Essentials for Certification. When the essentials went before the 1978 House, they were passed and the process was in motion.[9] The objectives of the 1978 essentials were divided into three sections:

1. **Patient care**:

The establishment of the specialty recognition was to

a. promote a high level of quality care,

b. assist the consumer in the identification of physical therapists with specialized clinical skill, and

c. ensure the present scope of practice of physical therapy and facilitate future development.

2. **Research**:

The process was to promote the development of the science-art underlying the profession of physical therapy.

3. **Education**:

The process was to

FIGURE 4-2
Commission Members—1978

Sandy Burkart	— Orthopaedics
Carolyn Crutchfield	— Neurology
Carolyn Heriza	— Pediatrics
Scot Irwin	— Cardiopulmonary
Patricia Sullivan	— Measurement Expert
Vernon Nickel, M.D.	— Consumer member
George Soper	— Board of Directors

---

a. provide assistance to the education systems in planning curriculum to develop specialists and

b. to improve communication with other professions.

The 1978 essentials also outlined an organizational structure that included a commission to oversee the process and specialty councils that would develop the certification process in each designated area. The entire process is under the auspices or directive of the House, which approves the formation of each specialty council only upon recommendation of the Commission for Certification of Advanced Clinical Competence (later called the Board for Certification of Advanced Clinical Competence and now called the American Board of Physical Therapy Specialties [ABPTS]).

In 1978, the commission was comprised of representatives from four specialty areas that were identified as having existing patterns of practice that most likely would constitute specialization in physical therapy (Fig.4-2). A rotation system now has been established for the speciality board so that all clinical areas with a certification process will have representation.

Nature and Dimensions of the Certification Process

Commission for Clinical Competence

The commission had the onerous task of accepting responsibility from the House for a goal that the Association had adopted relatively slowly and then wanted to see put into place and implemented immediately. The commission had its first meeting in 1979 and established its initial functions, which included establishing organizational structure, developing procedures to implement the essentials, identifying common areas of knowledge, developing the certificate and setting up data-management systems, and establishing fiscal guidelines. Some of these functions were put into place systematically and easily. Others have yet to be brought into fruition.

The commission had the choice either to develop a process that was defensible before specialty councils were formed or to establish a system that allowed specialty council involvement as the process was developed. The pressing need in some areas to provide credentials to verify the physical therapist's role in a particular area of care necessitated a relatively simultaneous process. This simultaneous process allowed greater freedom, in some respects, before the councils could propose various methods of accomplishing a task within the general guidelines of the essentials. This process also allowed for a variety of testing methodologies to be proposed and evaluated. However, this process also increased the risk that the proposed process would be examined by the commission, be found not to offer the necessary reliability and validity of process, and be rejected.

Specialty Process

The process has proceeded from these beginnings to one in 1988 where five areas have completed the administration of examinations under the auspices of the ABPTS, which include cardiopulmonary, electrophysiologic, neurology, pediatrics, and sports physical therapy. Orthopaedic physical therapy is expected to conduct its initial exam in 1989. The process has required careful scrutiny and preparation. A brief review of the process itself will allow a better understanding of what has been created and how well the profession's goals have been met.

Developing a Petition

The process is initiated by a group all of which up to this point have been sections of the APTA that believe their members practice at an advanced level of care. The major portion of work in developing a petition is to identify the knowledge and skills beyond entry level that delineate the advanced clinician or practice.[10] The groups petitioning are free to choose the method by which these are identified, and the documentation can include role delineation determined by a group of acknowledged experts (eg, Delphi study) or a job analysis through a survey of practice.

The competencies identified are to reflect observable behaviors of the clinician in a manner that requires a combination of knowledge, skills, and attitude necessary to practice in the specialty area. The competencies are to be presented in a manner so that the reader cannot only identify the competency (Fig.4-3), but also understand the spectrum of the competency by examples of conditions in which the competency is to be demonstrated (Fig.4-4), examples of learning experiences to attain or develop the competency (Fig.4-5), and examples of methods of evaluation (Fig.4-6). Each competency also is to have the rationale and evidence on which the competency is deemed advanced (Fig.4-7), in addition to the knowledge needed to perform the competency (Fig.4-8).

This structure assures that a number of premises of the essentials are fulfilled. These premises include that 1) there is an observable skill level, 2) the process does not require any one learning environment, 3) and that the competency has been documented as advanced or beyond entry level.

The spectrum of competencies, as outlined by the essentials, focuses on a broad skill and knowledge level within the specialty area. The competencies are to be placed under the following general headings of 1) patient examination; 2) planning, implementing, and evaluating programs of care as required by the specialty area; 3) interpretation of scientific literature and use of the research process; 4) teaching; and 5) communication.

FIGURE 4-3
Cardiopulmonary Competency I—Patient Care
Conducts a Patient Evaluation

G. Conducts or assists in conduction of definitive evaluation procedures and interprets patient data including but not limited to:
  graded exercise testing—low level or maximal functional capacity
  graded exercise testing with blood gas or expiratory air measurements
  measurements of inspiratory and expiratory pressures, volume and flow
  1. Selects method and instrumentation/equipment
     a) describes in detail the procedures and instrumentation employed for any normal test
     b) lists indication and contraindication of the test
  2. Prepares the patient for testing
     a) physically
     b) mentally
  3. Administers and records result of the test
     a) set and manipulate test instruments
     b) recognize, detect and record response to test procedure
     c) alleviate unnecessary discomfort
  4. Modifies or terminates the evaluative procedures, if necessary when the therapist determines the:
     a) patient's safety is compromised
     b) patient's discomfort exceeds levels necessary for procedure
     c) patient's cooperation is necessary and he/she is no longer able or willing to cooperate
     d) equipment becomes faulty
     e) procedure does not, or ceases to yield results necessary for evaluating patient's cardiopulmonary problems
     f) patient's safe physiologic response is compromised
     g) patient's financial limitations are prohibitive
  5. Interprets evaluative findings appropriately
     a) states and communicates the results of the evaluation
     b) relates the evaluative findings to the patient's:
         i. medical history
         ii. disease process
         iii. current medical treatment
         iv. presenting symptoms
         v. disease progression and stage of symptoms
         vi. present level of function
         vii. related diagnostic test finding
         viii. current medications
     c) establishes a course of action which may include:
         i. a physical therapy plan of care
         ii. referring the patient back to the physician
         iii. recommending to the physician other definitive procedures
         iv. consulting with other health care team members

CARDIOPULMONARY PHYSICAL THERAPY ADVANCED CLINICAL COMPETENCIES 1983

FIGURE 4-4
Neurology Physical Therapy Competency I:
Conduct an Initial Screening on a Patient with
a Neurologic Deficit

Example of Conditions
1. Given a patient with a neurologic deficit, for example, closed head injury, hemiplegia, Parkinson's Disease, cerebellar deficit, spinal cord injury, cerebral palsy.
2. A 22-year-old man, living with his parents, was referred to a rehabilitation hospital that is located 4 hours from his home. At the age of 14 he had sustained a right mandibular, right femoral and right humeral fracture as well as a traumatic head injury resulting in a coma lasting two months. The referral material containing the past medical history is complete regarding surgical procedures, but scanty regarding cognitive, motor and functional performance. He is to be assessed by the physician and physical therapist in 20 to 30 minutes at an outpatient clinic visit to determine the need for inpatient rehabilitation services, consultative services or referral to services within the local community.

NEUROLOGIC PHYSICAL THERAPY ADVANCED CLINICAL COMPETENCIES 1985

FIGURE 4-5
Pediatric Physical Therapy
Competency 7: Individual Education Plan (IEP)

Example of Learning Experiences

Learning experiences leading to independent skill may include the following:
1. Development of knowledge base in clinical sciences, kinesiology, physiology, behavioral sciences, normal growth and sensorimotor development, through didactic training, either of a formal or informal nature.
2. Development of knowledge base of PL 94-142, with appropriate state implementing "Rules and Regulations."
3. Development of knowledge base of appropriate pediatric assessment(s) and program planning for children with developmental disabilities, birth defects, neuromuscular musculoskeletal defects (i.e., cerebral palsy, myelodysplasia, developmental delay, muscular dystrophy, cardiopulmonary dysfunction).
4. Observation of instructional audio-visual materials of assessment(s) techniques and program planning, including written behavioral goals and objectives, of children with various developmental disabilities.
5. Administration and interpretation of appropriate assessment(s), including program planning, on actual children with developmental disabilities, with and without supervision.

In 3, 4 and 5 above, the learner will:
a. Administer appropriate pediatric assessment(s).
b. Determine need for intervention and/or referral.
c. Formulate appropriate student annual goals and short term objectives as indicated by assessment.
d. Design an appropriate physical therapy management plan, consistent with student's educational goals.
e. Participate in formulating the IEP and determining program placement.

PEDIATRICS PHYSICAL THERAPY ADVANCED CLINICAL COMPETENCIES 1985

FIGURE 4-6
Clinical Electrophysiologic Physical Therapy
Competency I: Patient Care

Example of Evaluation:
 1. Written objective tests on neuromuscular electrophysiology, instrumentation and quantification of EMG signals.
 2. Given a hypothetical patient situation, therapist will describe rationale for procedure, method of kinesiologic EMG analysis and implication of findings.

CLINICAL ELECTROPHYSIOLOGY PHYSICAL THERAPY ADVANCED CLINICAL COMPETENCIES 1985

FIGURE 4-7
Clinical Electrophysiologic Physical Therapy
Competency I: Patient Care

Rationale for Advanced Competence:

 Based on criteria established by the Clinical Electrophysiologic Specialty Council, these items in the competency validation survey were rated high in importance as advanced competencies, and therefore require examination in the cognitive domain.

CLINICAL ELECTROPHYSIOLOGY PHYSICAL THERAPY ADVANCED CLINICAL COMPETENCIES 1984

The petition also is to include a "map" of all outlined competencies, which allows the reader to have an overview of the advanced practice (Fig.4-9).

Designation/Function of Specialty Councils

After the petition is accepted, the ABPTS appoints a Specialty Council.[11] The very success of the certification process rests with this small group of three. The council's responsibilities are numerous. Their goal is to complete a process that results in specialists being certified by the ABPTS.

What is this group responsible for? They must validate the competencies presented in the petition (based on evidence that the competencies are advanced, necessary, and practiced by clinicians in the field); they must establish criteria (under the general guidelines provided by the ABPTS) to sit for the examination and a method to evaluate documentation provided to meet the criteria; they must decide how to test for clinical competencies in a multiple choice format (use of case studies) that tests all competencies designated; they must conduct item writing workshops to achieve a large enough item bank to create an exam; they must construct the exam (including a designated percentage of questions for each competency); and they must set a passing score. They then review the test results and recommend to the ABPTS who should be certified.

FIGURE 4-8
Sports Physical Therapy Competency II: Recognize
Dermatologic, Infectious and Medical Problems of the Athlete

Knowledge Needed to Perform Competency:

1. Anatomy
   a) Musculoskeletal
   b) Circulatory
   c) Cardiopulmonary
   d) Neurological
   e) Renal
   f) Urogenital
   g) Dental
   h) Visual
2. Physiology
   a) Musculoskeletal
   b) Circulatory
   c) Cardiopulmonary
   d) Neurological
   e) Renal
   f) Urogenital
   g) Dental
   h) Visual
3. Understanding the etiology of dermatologic, medical, and infectious problems.
4. Psychology
   a) Emotional response of athlete to dermatologic, infectious, and general medical problems.
5. Sociology
   a) Families' influence on athlete suffering from medical, dermatologic, and infectious disorders.
6. Pharmacology
   a) Actions and reactions of drugs and medications.
7. Observation
   a) Ability to recognize dermatologic, infectious, and medical athletic problems.
8. Administration
   a) Modification of equipment or uniform to minimize further exacerbation of dermatologic, infectious, or medical problems.
   b) Counsel the athlete regarding a change in personal habits and hygiene.
   c) Refer to appropriate medical specialist

SPORTS PHYSICAL THERAPY ADVANCED CLINICAL COMPETENCIES 1985

Designation/Function of the American Board of Physical Therapy Specialties

The members of the ABPTS representing clinical specialties are appointed by the ABPTS and serve a four-year term.[9] The clinical measurements or testing experts appointment also is made by the ABPTS. The APTA Board of Directors member and the consumer member are appointed by the APTA Board.

The ABPTS has the broad task of 1) accepting a petition; 2) appointing

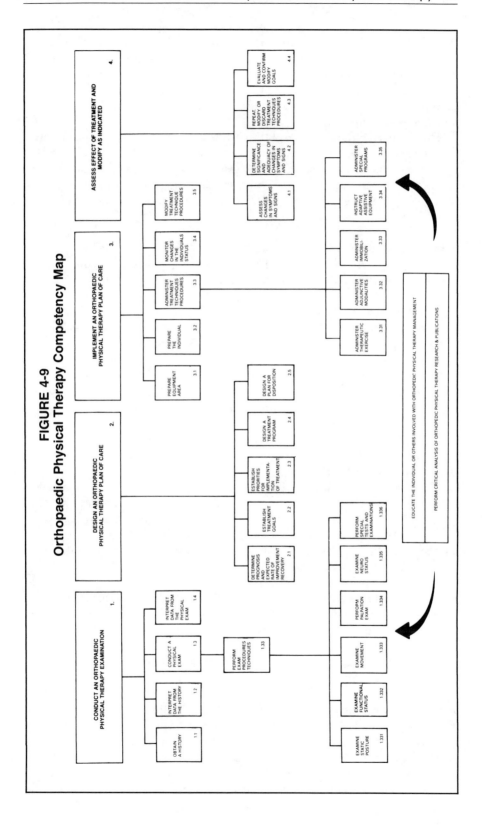

FIGURE 4-9
Orthopaedic Physical Therapy Competency Map

council members after presenting the petition to the House; 3) establishing guidelines and policies for certification development within the framework of the essentials; 4) reviewing proposed criteria, review processes, examination-development, and examinationdelivery modes of the councils; 5) evaluating examination results; 6) certifying qualified individuals; and 7) achieving financial independence.

The financial independence of the certification process will not be possible until larger numbers have completed the examination. It is a credit to the profession that the House of Delegates and Board of Directors, APTA, continue their support of expenditures to allow the process to proceed. The review of expenditures and creation of a system that allows financial independence is a goal of the ABPTS.

Policies/Procedures of Process

Within the duties of the ABPTS, the following policies and procedures have been developed as basic criteria for specialty certification.

Competencies. The competencies for each specialty area, once validated and accepted by the ABPTS, are to be published for potential candidates. The competencies must be revalidated every 10 years.

Examination. Eligibility criteria to sit for the initial examination in any specialty area are stringent. The initial minimal criteria include the following:
1. Six thousand hours of documented clinical time in the specialty area, all of which must be within the last ten years.
2. Written evidence of competency in administration and communication; education; and research.
3. Three character references.

The eligibility focus is on clinical expertise; however, the essentials also require that those certified have skills in the areas of communication (administration), education, and research. The initial criteria to sit for the examination requires documentation and review of competency in these areas before admission to the written examination. As the process continues to develop, these criteria are subject to revision.

Examination Development. The ABPTS has determined that each council is to work with a designated testing agency.[11] Each council may develop processes that are unique to its needs, within the capabilities of the testing agency. This means that the council may propose and initiate its own item writing workshop, but that the final items must be in a format acceptable to the testing agency.

Item Development. The development of items is done through input from and work of clinicians active in the particular area of practice. The criteria to be an item writer are set by the council and approved by the ABPTS.

The items must be a multiple-choice construct, but they may be centered around case studies. A number of councils have used the case study format successfully in developing multiple-choice questions that can indicate candidates' evaluative and judgment skills in addition to their level of knowledge. This ability to test for evaluation and judgment skills, of course, is important in delineating clinical specialists.

Examination Construction. Each council must match items to the validated competencies and design an examination that tests all competencies.[11] This process must include a review of all items and use of expert judgment in establishing the level of the test item (eg, the test item tests at knowledge level that is essential to know or the test item tests at a judgment level and is essential to know) (Fig. 4-10).

Designation of Certified Individuals. The council, in conjunction with the testing agency, must establish a passing score for the examination. They then must present the process of establishing the passing score, the actual passing score, and candidate test results to the ABPTS. The ABPTS then credentials as specialists those who satisfactorily complete the requirements.

Examination Alternatives Including Orals or Practicals. The process at this time has designated minimal guidelines for oral or practical examinations. The process currently does not require use of either oral or practical examination, and the initiation of their use in the future will be through a council demonstrating a need to use an oral or practical to test the clinician adequately.

Recertification. The speciality process includes recertification that must occur within seven years of the initial certification.[12] Various models and methods may be used. The focus will be on a reasonable process that does not require more stringent criteria than for sitting for the initial examination.

Subspecialization. The process of specialty certification has proceeded to subspecialty certification in other professions, most notably in medicine.[13] The specialty certification process in physical therapy currently has no method of establishing subspecialty areas.

Financial Independence. The initial criteria of 1975 stated financial independence as a goal for the specialization process.[7] The recognition of the complexity of the process to develop certification has resulted in the House passing a motion in 1986 that allows for continued funding of ABPTS functions.[14] Each council is responsible for its own expenses, and, to date, these have been provided through section support.

Future Directions

In 1985, the first three specialists were certified in cardiopulmonary physical therapy. Not only are these initial three specialists a credit to themselves and the profession, but they also are a credit to the people who designed and materialized the process. On February 12, 1987, the first official recognition ceremony for specialists was held at the Combined Sections Meeting in Atlanta, Georgia. At this ceremony, twelve more specialists were

FIGURE 4-10
Excerpt from Validation Survey
Cardiopulmonary Specialty Council 1986

1. Frequency of Performance

    Very Frequently   Frequently   Occasionally   Never

2. Importance

    Essential   Desirable   Not Essential/Not Desirable

3. Level

    Basic   Advanced

F. Conduct evaluation including but not limited to:

1. Physical Examination

    a. inspection: Observation
       rate, rhythm, pattern of
       breathing, ventilatory muscle use
       thoracic cage symmetry
       spinal curvature
       AP: Lat diameter
       skin; color
       extremities; edema, clubbing

    b. palpation:
       neck
       thoracic cage
       subcostal angle
       expansion, excursion
       peripheral pulses

    c. percussion

    d. auscultation:
       breath sounds

certified: five in cardiopulmonary; four in pediatrics; and three in electrophysiologic physical therapy. As of 1988, there are 78 board certified specialists.

Board Certified Specialist-Ramification

These questions often are asked: What has this process created? Is this board certified specialist functioning differently than the noncertified board "specialist"? Is this process simply self-aggrandizement? These questions are not easy to answer and will remain difficult to respond to until a larger number of therapists are certified.

The criteria to sit for the initial examination have been stringent, and a review of the clinicians who currently are board certified finds a group who already were practicing in positions that required advanced skill. It therefore is difficult to state that the potential for particular positions has improved or changed dramatically by becoming certified. These individuals, however, now hold credentials that will assume increased meaning when competing for a position advertised as a clinical specialist position.

The speciality process, nonetheless, offers more than increased advantage in the employment market. The primary benefit and focus of this process is in clinical skill or care delivered to the patient or consumer. This process provides a verification or substantiation to the consumer that the clinician is expert in a particular field of practice. This expertise therefore should benefit the consumer in the same way that board certification can benefit the consumer when in need of thoracic surgery or internal medicine. For example, this process may lead the consumer to seek a particular practitioner according to present complaints or disorders. It also provides the consumer with outside verification of the clinician's own claim to expertise in a special area.

Additionally, I believe this process will assume other manifestations of the medical specialty system. I believe, for example, that the board certified individual will be used increasingly as a consultant to other clinicians who may not have dealt as extensively in a particular field or with a specific disability. This use of the consultant will cross boundaries of a particular institution or environment. This occurs now but not at the frequency or consistency that I believe would benefit both the consumer and the profession. I also believe that the specialist, therefore, will become a tertiary care deliverer. Not only may the noncertified practitioner consult with the specialist but may believe that it is in the best interest to the client to be referred to the specialist for direct intervention. This referral will not hinder the general practitioner but will assist in networking, which will allow the optimum care for the difficult or complicated patient.

Importance to the Profession

Is this speciality process good for the profession? Is this potentially providing a divisive force? Is this a grand scheme to help a few and possibly harm others? The questions posed are critical to the process and are real. The profession is a broad one, spanning every age group and disability. The very existence of the sections in the Association demonstrates the desire of professionals practicing with a focus on similar areas of care to meet, share, and learn from each other. The complexity of patient problems and the technological advances in health care, in general, have expanded the scope of practice, knowledge, and skill in the profession beyond the imagination of even twenty years ago.

We not only are in need of a broad spectrum of clinicians with individual skills but of documentation that what is practiced daily actually assists in the rehabilitation of the client. The board certified specialist must show evidence of knowledge and understanding of the research process. These individuals are the persons in the profession to whom we should look for the research to validate our practice. Even if the number remains seemingly small, the impact that these individuals can make on our profession can be great and important to our growth.

Future Sights

I believe that this specialty process will cross national and international borders. Clinicians from other countries have written already inquiring if they are eligible to sit for an examination. The criteria are written broadly (eg, eligible to belong to the APTA, with a background of equivalent training) to allow for the eventual sitting of therapists from other countries. Additionally, the World Confederation for Physical Therapy endorsed the concept of board certification in specialty areas in 1982.[15]

I am hopeful that we will continue to use our knowledge and experience well and to foster the growth of the process of certification, using the insights of our mistakes and the focus of optimum care for the client.

References
1. Wellington E: Physiotherapy in general hospital practice. Physther Rev. 7(3): 8-12, 1927.
2. Stewart HE: Educational requirements of the present and future in physiotherapy. Physther Rev. 7(3): 3-5, 1927.
3. Courses for graduates at Harvard Medical School. Physther Rev. 7(2): 30, 1927.
4. McMillan M: Lower back conditions. Physther Rev. 7(2): 24-30, 1927.
5. Crutchfield C: Specialization: Its current status. Clinical Management in Physical Therapy. 4(5), 38-39, 1984.
6. RC 20-73: Specialization in physical therapy. In: House of Delegates Minutes. Alexandria, VA, American Physical Therapy Association, 1973.
7. RC 16-75: APTA policy statement on recognition of specialists in physical therapy. In: House of Delegates Minutes. Alexandria, VA, American Physical Therapy Association, 1975.
8. RC 32-75: Task Force on clinical specialization. In: House of Delegates Minutes. Alexandria, VA, American Physical Therapy Association, 1975.
9. RC 30-78: Essentials for certification of physical therapy specialties. In: House of Delegates Minutes. Alexandria, VA, American Physical Therapy Association 1978.

10. Instructions for completion of a petition to establish a specialty area. In: Policy and Procedure Manual: American Board of Physical Therapy Specialties. Alexandria, VA, American Physical Therapy Association, 1986.
11. Examination. In: Policy and Procedure Manual: American Board of Physical Therapy Specialties. Alexandria, VA, American Physical Therapy Association, 1986.
12. Recertification. In: Policy and Procedure Manual: American Board of Physical Therapy Specialties. Alexandria, VA, American Physical Therapy Association, 1986.
13. Subspecialization. In: Policy and Procedure Manual: American Board of Physical Therapy Specialties, Alexandria, VA, American Physical Therapy Association, 1986.
14. RC 10-86: Recognition of Specialists in Physical Therapy. In: House of Delegates Minutes. Alexandria, VA, CA, American Physical Therapy Association, 1986 p. 9.
15. Minute: Guidelines on Specialization. In: Minutes of the General Meeting. London, England, World Confederation for Physical Therapy, 1982.

CHAPTER 5

Physical Therapists Assistant Issues in the 1980s and 1990s

Cheryl Webster Carpenter, CPTA

A review of the history of the creation of the physical therapist will be helpful in understanding the role of the assistant in physical therapy and in the APTA.

During the 1960s, a big push occurred by the government to initiate health care training programs at the junior college level. Interest grew regarding the field of physical therapy, and a prediction was made about the potential for shortages as the field grew.[11] An assistant to fill the void in this field could be of great value in the future. The creation of assistants was not meant to relieve the physical therapist of professional duties but was meant to transfer tasks that could be delegated safely to supportive personnel. That would allow the use of physical therapists in those areas that cannot be delegated. The junior colleges approached the American Physical Therapy Association to develop guidelines regarding the assistant's training at that level. In 1965, the APTA House of Delegates resolved that an ad hoc committee be formed specifically to study the utilization and training of nonprofessional assistants. The charge was completed in 1967 when the House adopted the Policy Statement on the Training and the Utilization of the Physical Therapy Assistant.[1]

In 1967, the House adopted the formal policy statement regarding the Training and Utilization of physical therapist assistants. Along with the policy statement, a mandate for the following was established: 1) that the APTA was to establish the standards for the program, which also meant an attendant process of some form of accreditation; 2) that a supervisory relationship should exist between the physical therapist and the assistant; 3) that the functions of the assistant should be identified; 4) that mandatory licensure or registration, incorporated into existing physical therapy laws, should be encouraged; and 5) that a category of membership be established in the APTA for the physical therapist assistant.[1]

After the policy statement was adopted, the APTA Board of Directors appointed the Task Force on Supportive Personnel. This task force developed guidelines for the training and use of the physical therapist assistant.[3,4]

In 1973, the Affiliate membership class was established for the physical therapist assistant. Heated debate over this issue took place because a non-professional was gaining membership into a professional organization. During the five years it took to prepare for this new category of membership, the APTA had kept the membership informed of developments and had moved with the times. Although controversy existed within the membership, the action would have implications for the enhancing the future of physical therapy.

Current Issues

Since the creation and evolution of the physical therapist assistant, physical therapists have expressed feeling threatened, at the practice level, by the perception that assistants would one day take over the therapist's role. This concept has been deemed ill-founded on the basis of the supervisory relationship found in clinics and the importance of the supervisory relationship so often stressed in physical therapist assistant education programs.[8]

The perceived problem could stem from the lack of communication between physical therapists and physical therapist assistants. Unfortunately, poor communication does not promote a workable practice. This problem accentuates the misconception that the physical therapist assistant will usurp the role of the physical therapist, making the perceived situation much worse than it is in reality.

Formally trained physical therapist assistants, from day one, have been influenced by physical therapists: the physical therapist assistant program directors and faculty. The attitudes the directors display can create a healthy base from which to grow in relationship to the profession and to the assistants' role. Unfortunately, once assistants are out of school, their opportunities for growth may not be visible to them. Physical therapists often are unsure how to use assistants, delegating cleaning, secretarial, and other inappropriate activities that unfortunately are neither motivating nor suitable to the assistant graduate. Nonetheless, these are the types of duties assigned sometimes to assistants in clinical situations. An assistant probably will not stay long in this type of practice, and a quick departure itself can leave a bad impression with a therapist.

Appropriate use of assistants can be a positive experience for all parties involved from therapists to administrators of hospitals. The use of physical therapist assistants is a cost-effective measure. In most states, physical therapists usually can supervise two to three physical therapist assistants. This is not to say that physical therapist assistants can replace the activities of physical therapists, but they can carry out programs developed and supervised by physical therapists, thereby enabling therapists to perform evaluative, administrative, and research oriented activities. Many therapists have expressed the belief that their direct patient contact is jeopardized by allowing an assistant to treat patients. In a healthy balance, the opposite is true: two pairs of eyes are better than one, and both can learn from each other if the mind is open.

What is the appropriate utilization of the assistant? The APTA long ago established guidelines that give therapists an outline. Unfortunately, those guidelines do not always solve or prevent clinical problems. Intuition and common sense, for example, can be keys to understanding individual capabilities. Assistants cannot be left without supervision and be expected to survive. Working with an assistant is a process of communicating and learning about each others strengths and weaknesses. Physical therapists frequently state, "My clinic is just not set up to employ physical therapist assistants." But after listening to their viewpoints, you often find their concepts about work assignments contrary to what assistants are capable of doing. As cost-effectiveness becomes essential in health care, assistants will be employed in an increasing number of clinical settings.

Education

Many physical therapists have said to assistants, "If you want to practice as a physical therapist, go back to school and obtain your degree." Many assistants, however, enjoy being physical therapist assistants and all that the position entails. Unfortunately, this viewpoint of therapists does not allow for focusing on and enhancing the individual strengths of their assistant.

Issues raised over the choice of an educational program should be closely examined. Many persons who enter an assistant program may have the intellectual capacity to become a physical therapist but are not able to do so. Reasons expressed to the author include time or money constraints and location of a physical therapy program in relation to home and family commitments.

For those assistants who have returned to educational settings to obtain a degree in physical therapy, many have found their assistants' coursework cannot be transferred. Although many of them have learned modality application as assistants, they cannot be given credit for that. This lack of credit can be a significant disappointment to students and make them feel unrecognized for their education and skills as assistants. The option should be left to the individuals and based on their previous education and practical experiences. From early reports of this issue, educators and clinicians tended to agree with the necessity for educational advancement opportunities for the physical therapist assistants.[1,4,6]

Proliferation of Physical Therapist Assistant Programs

The number of school administrators indicating an interest in creating assistant programs has been on the rise in the past two decades. As physical therapy professional education continues to advance to the postbaccalaureate degree level, physical therapist assistants will become an alternative to personnel shortages. Although it is suggested that the requirement of a postbaccalaureate degree will not add to the shortage dilemma, it appears that money, opportunity for growth, and research funds, will influence the job market in attracting people. These benefits have not always been available to physical therapists and with numerous cutbacks in funding at many facilities these opportunities will become less available.

Physical therapist assistant programs currently are receiving applicants beyond their enrollment capabilities. New programs will help to meet the needs of those unable to gain entrance into existing assistant programs. A concern sometimes expressed is that many assistants do not relocate after graduation, but the physical therapy needs of most communities especially rural, are large enough to promote the creation of an assistant program in a local junior college and guarantee jobs to the graduates.

Many of the new programs for assistants are in states that currently do not have physical therapist assistant programs or state laws that define the assistant's role and scope of practice. New programs in those states will encourage chapters to seek legislation regulating the practice of the assistant at the state level.

Time will continue to demonstrate the need for upgrading the standards of education for the physical therapist assistant. As the physical therapy profession advances, physical therapist assistant programs will feel the push toward progressive studies in all aspects of physical therapy.

Licensure or Certification

In the future of physical therapist assistants, licensure or certification will continue to be essential.[2] One question to ponder is, "What does the physical therapist assistant in unregulated states do in practice?" The answer often is "we are unsure." It is important to recognize the potential for consumer abuse from assistants in such unregulated states. How does the consumer in the current system know which physical therapy services are to be rendered by a physical therapist (eg, evaluation) and which are to be rendered by the physical therapist assistant? Other than insurance requirements in those states that do not have assistant regulation, a physical therapist assistant is not required by law to be supervised or directed. Physical therapist assistant legislation would offer consumer protection to the potential physical therapy patient. Additionally, legislation would define for therapists their responsibilities and prohibit a potential entrepreneurial abuse situation of using assistants for a profitable gain by the therapist-owner (ie, having one therapist supervise more than two to three assistants at a time).

This example is not to be misconstrued as saying the delineation of supervision has to be so strict as not to allow assistants to practice without direct on-site supervision. Supervision is dependent upon the capabilities of the assistants and the structure of the facility.

For reimbursement purposes, physical therapist assistants' roles and job differentiation will need to be defined. Does this responsibility rest with physical therapists or physical therapist assistants? Both parties should shoulder the task to reach a solution that will be amiable and comfortable to all parties.

Most physical therapist assistants are willing to work within the constraints of their training and often are anxious to become involved politically to accomplish licensure or certification. Physical therapist assistant program administrators should be activists in the legislative arena. The people who graduate from the programs sometimes are unaware of the licensure or certification requirements in other states and often are surprised when relocating to a state that does require such credentials.

Personnel Shortages

As the profession of physical therapy continues to grow and its population grows older, new areas of practice will emerge that require physical therapy services.[7] A great opportunity lies ahead for all persons in physical therapy with innovative ideas. Unfortunately, the growth in patient-client populations does not necessarily mean that the professional work force will be able to meet the demand. As initially identified in 1962, personnel shortages will continue to exist. If physical therapists and physical therapist assistants are not available to meet the demand, someone else will; then it will be too late to have control over the situation. This problem is somewhat commonplace now. In the event a physical therapist or physical therapist assistant is not available to carry out services, a person who often is on-the-job trained or who is untrained will provide physical therapy. This does not necessarily mean the treatment is billed as such a service-but it means no control is exercised over the person rendering the treatment. This scenario, of course, does not mention the potential danger to the patient. This lack of appropriately trained staff is prevalent in rural areas currently. If there is a potential for physical therapists to contract their services to a setting and for physical therapist assistants to be available to carry out the treatment outlined by physical therapists, more of an acceptable treatment can be delivered to the patient. In this situation, the assistant has the obligation to the therapist and to the patient to ensure the treatment will be carried out in an appropriate manner.

Advancement Opportunities

It appears odd for a profession not to encourage development within its own field for assistants. At some point in time, it will be necessary to give credit to assistants and advance them within the current structure, whether it be in the Association or in educational or clinical settings.

Opportunities for development exist for assistants within the physical therapy or physical therapist assistant programs. Potential exists for participating in lectures, laboratory instruction, and other educational opportunities. Assistants often are qualified by their experience and interest in a specified area, whether it be of a clinical or research orientation.

If an assistant, for instance, is quite talented in an area such as quality assurance, where is it written that a physical therapist assistant cannot participate in this project? Candidates entering physical therapist assistant programs may already have a bachelor's or a master's degree. In such cases, there should be no reason to penalize a person secondary to their job title or description, that could mean another case of not utilizing a physical therapist assistant appropriately.

Job satisfaction for assistants is currently under study. Early results have been included in a study from the University of Alabama at Birmingham reported in a poster presentation at the APTA 1988 Annual Conference. The implications of the study in relation to employment setting and geographical location will be helpful to employers and physical therapy assistant program directors.

Currently, few facilities offer positions for advancement. Research is currently being done at various facilities on this issue. At some time, opportunity for advancement may be commonplace to enhance assistants to stay at a facility once they have gained essential expertise for that facility. Physical therapists have a tendency not to stay at the same acute care setting more than two to three years after graduation from entry-level programs. Assistants can lend stability to a facility and can educate and provide inservice for newcomers to the clinics existing programs and policies. Too often, assistants are self-limited by their titles. They do not realize their potential and do not exercise their creativeness. Opportunities for advancement are not handed to assistants, they have to have ingenuity and drive to create and use them.

Specialization

As therapists move toward specialization within the field, so will assistants. Many conditions treated demand special expertise. To provide the best possible treatment to some patients, assistants will need to specialize. This often means advanced training that is not currently offered to them. Many seminars and workshops are limited to enrollment solely by physical therapists. The APTA is beginning to offer opportunities for continuing education for the assistant.

Physical therapist assistants, just as physical therapists, are expected to participate in continuing-education courses to stay abreast of new technologies in the field. As research becomes more of a focus by many therapists, assistants will be expected to be consumers of research and apply new concepts, based on their supervising therapists' evaluations.

Evaluation skills of assistants will require refinement. A physical therapist assistant must evaluate all patients before rendering the treatment protocol set by a physical therapist on any given treatment day. All patients do not progress; some even may regress between treatment sessions, so the assistant must be aware of the changes. The realization that assistants do evaluate will continue to cause controversy, but this evolution is necessary in the progressive field of physical therapy.

Association Membership

Attempts are being made currently to increase the involvement of the assistant as affiliate members at the Association level. It is important to note that the early development of affiliate membership for assistants is paralleled to that of active membership for physical therapists in the infancy of the APTA. The nurturing and encouragement of involvement in the Association by the APTA is a healthy relationship. Many affiliate members would like to become involved more actively in the Association but do not find the opportunity, just as many active members would like to become more involved at a national level.

When the Organizational Structure Task Force[5] has completed work for presentation to the 1989 House, it will be hard to project what over 400 delegates will decide to establish as the structure of the future Association compared with how it is known today. Some active members have expressed concern at the suggestion of aligning nonprofessionals with professionals in an association such as the APTA. However, problems in physical therapy often brought forth to the House affect therapists and assistants at all levels when policies are put into effect. House of Delegates decisions regarding practice, for example, can have an overall effect on all physical therapy practitioners manner of practice. When the policies are scrutinized by governmental agencies, insurance companies, or the general public, the APTA is looked at as the expert in the field of physical therapy.

Issues of how the assistants should be used are brought to the House and decided by the physical therapists who are delegates because they greatly outnumber the assistants who are delegates. Assistants' comments regarding impending policy changes rarely are sought prior to presentation of the proposed policy to the House. Physical therapists should realize, however, that they are ultimately responsible for the actions of physical therapist assistants and they should allow assistants to make some decisions regarding their modes of practice.

Although the past voting trends of Affiliates in the House are not trackable at this time, a number of previous delegates believe the Affiliates have voted in the majority and often have been directed delegates of their chapter on controversial issues.

Apportionment in the House has been identified as a major area of concern to active members. The number of affiliate members in the Association is less than that of the active members. The question than is: "Is it fair for active members to be penalized by not having as many active delegates when the affiliate membership in some states may be considerably smaller, in proportion?" If the membership will realize that the number of affiliate members at this time in the APTA is proportionate to the number of active members in membership during the formation of the Association, the current proportionment is fair. Active pursuit of Affiliate-Affiliate Student membership has not been a strong suit of the APTA, as pointed out in the results of the 1987 American Society of Association Executives' evaluation.[10] Should this proportionment stay the same over the next few years? The next five years should lend a new wave of affiliate members and subsequent involvement in the APTA. The affiliate member always should be allowed in the House, with a voice and a vote.

If the Affiliate Assembly concept[5] is adopted by the House, Affiliate delegates will provide for the Affiliate member input nationally and the affiliate delegates at the chapter level will continue to represent their state's assistants. As affiliate membership increases, a look at reapportionment may be in order. The Affiliate Assembly can be identified as means of increasing Affiliate membership and of providing the opportunity for Affiliate involvement that is at an appropriate level.

Suffice it to say, affiliate members should and will be a part of the Association in as much as they still are an integral part of the physical therapy profession. As long as physical therapists and physical therapist assistants intertwine in practice, many issues will face both groups that will demand mutual exchange.

Since 1983, communication between the Affiliate Special Interest Group (ASIG) and the APTA has been on the rise and will continue to be facilitated by both groups, which is a positive step by the Association. Communication is the key to understanding for both groups. Many people are unsure of the relationship of the ASIG to the APTA and how each stands to benefit. Because the focus of the Association remains on physical therapy, issues of working together for a common goal will clarify the means. The level of involvement in the Association the Affiliate member may seek will depend on the opportunities that exist. The Association and its membership often fail to realize the type of input Affiliate members have to offer. In many physical therapist assistant programs, much centers around the fact that physical therapists and physical therapist assistants are a team, a team that heavily relies on each member for input to aid in the optimum result of physical therapy. Relationships at the Association level can benefit from the same type of input.

Involvement at a national level will continue to be input oriented, but should begin at least to be product oriented, mandating the generation of reports and studies by PTA's. Research regarding assistants' practices, utilization, continuing-education opportunities, and employment potential should be delegated to physical therapist assistants. The Foundation of Physical Therapy could support that research. This is not an innovative idea. Assistants in the field are doing research and writing articles. Some have appeared in *Clinical Management in Physical Therapy* and other Association publications.

At the Association level, some recognition must be made of physical therapist assistants for accomplishments within their own area. Advancements made by assistants often go unnoticed by the profession as a whole. These advances may not be as monumental as those made by physical therapists, but they are noteworthy to their peers.

Affiliate Special Interest Group

In 1983, the Florida Chapter presented a motion to the House to form a section for the affiliate member to address the special concerns and interest of the affiliate. The motion was declined by the House, but within the same session the Affiliate Special Interest Group was created as an informal ad hoc group not defined in the Bylaws but recognized by and encouraged by the APTA Board.

The ASIG met after the 1983 House session and began to formalize a group in which the affiliate and student affiliate members' concerns could be addressed. Means of organization were defined in their Rules and Regulations[9] and officers were elected. Physical therapist assistant Regional Coordinators were appointed to inform the affiliate-affiliate student membership of the organization and the future plans. The baseline philosophy was to establish communication between the affiliate-affiliate student membership and the APTA Board of Directors to meet the special needs and interests of their membership.

The ASIG continues to serve in the capacity of liaison and will become the Affiliate Assembly if that concept is adopted by the 1989 House. The Affiliate Assembly, which has been mentioned briefly in this document, is defined by the author as an assembly in which affiliate and affiliate student members of the APTA would come together to promote interests and needs of that portion of the APTA membership. The outcome of the input, would be provided to the Board that would direct requests to the appropriate staff or departments for fulfillment within the APTA objectives. The Affiliate Assembly would never be considered a "Mini-House of Delegates." Affiliates desire the co-decision making process as currently available in the House.

The Affiliate Assembly may have two delegates to the House with one vote. The author believes that the Affiliate Assembly should be alloted delegates based on the proportion of affiliates on a nationwide basis. This truly would "serve" the needs of all affiliate members and at some point allow the removal of the affiliate delegate at the chapter level. Limited numbers of delegates in the Affiliate Assembly as outlined in Scenario Al will prohibit proportional representation of membership. Because affiliate members' salaries never will be commensurate with those of active members, decreased membership dues should be offered continually to affiliate members.[5]

Future Implications

Concerns over direct access for physical therapists also will affect physical therapist assistants in regard to practice. Physical therapists will require more concerted time for evaluation. Physical therapist assistants, therefore, will become more valuable to therapists in rendering the treatment programs designed by these therapist. Assistants will require not only more continuing education to stay abreast of new developments in the field but accelerated rates of PTA program coursework, to benefit the practice of therapists. This situation may bring an opportunity for advanced practice by assistants in certain practice settings. What the practice entails will be left to the individual therapist and assistant. Definition of the PTA work assignments may avoid problems with reimbursement that might exist if the nature of the work is not defined. Advanced practice may demand legislative action on issues of mandatory credentialing that need to be addressed on a state-by-state level. Assistants, for example, may need to be certified, registered, or licensed to be recognized by third party payers. Dissolution of grandfather clauses in state law, which allow on the job trained physical therapy aides to qualify to sit for the State's professional examination, will be essential for meeting reimbursement requirements. Questions regarding who is providing the service and their credentials will be asked.

In the future, what will be the plight of hospitals if they do not find innovative means by which to employ physical therapists? With less pay, decreased continuing education monies, and declining benefits currently in the offing, hospitals may become staffed primarily with assistants as employees and only with the minimum number of physical therapists to meet supervision requirements in the State law. If hospitals could market themselves and attract rehabilitation employees, they could become nationally renowned rehabilitation centers that not only offer the best in research, practice, and education for the professional but provide such services for the public and consumer. Specialized institutions that deal with specific diagnoses will continue to proliferate. Many of these institutions will be owned by companies not related to rehabilitation, but a professional atmosphere will be the primary mode of attracting clients. Staffing will be kept to a minimum and be advanced as the client population demands. At the hospital level, the use of diagnostic related groups will continue to force the discharge of patients at an accelerated pace. Governmental agencies will continue to place restrictions on home health agencies in an effort to ensure that high caliber care is provided. The need for skilled personnel will continue to rise, and assistants, therefore, will be used as a source of cost-containment. Issues of how independent assistants should be in the home health setting will be addressed continually.

Members' involvement in the Association activities will be based on the individual's qualifications for the responsibilities that are assumed in a job; therefore, it is essential that the APTA involve a mixture of members with various backgrounds and levels of expertise. Too often, the APTA does not offer certain individuals a chance for involvement and, thus, misses the opportunity for receiving innovative feedback. Currently the most comfortable mechanism for the involvement of the affiliate member in the Association is through the ASIG. This group serves as a training ground for affiliate members to become acquainted with the Association and its policies; additionally, it will develop leaders among affiliate members and groom them for appropriate roles within the Association. At some time, it would be beneficial to employ an affiliate member on the staff at APTA headquarters. This action would allow an affiliate member to answer questions throughout the day and to aid in the future legislative issues concerning affiliate members. Legislation that will define the practice of the physical therapy assistant is important.

Although provisions in physical therapist assistant programs to have additional positions for applicants will enable more people to become physical therapist assistants, special caution should be exercised to promote the fact that the assistant programs are not a stepping stone to physical therapy programs that lead to qualification as a physical therapist. This erroneous information has produced applicants who are unable to gain entrance into the physical therapy schools and, therefore, become assistants as a second choice. Physical therapist assistant program directors should be aware of this misconception and keep this in mind when they interview applicants.

If anyone should be threatened by the advancement of physical therapy assistants, it rightfully should be physical therapy aides who are trained on the job. Physical therapy aides have been allowed to provide physical therapy procedures under the supervision of the physical therapist. Now they may be relegated to providing only nonpatient related activities. Technicians who have been providing advanced treatment also will feel an effect on their job tasks because of the physical therapist assistant. This is a double-sided issue, however, because physical therapist assistants have a job status and are at a pay level that usually makes it inappropriate to delegate nonpatient related duties. In the future, however, we will see the physical therapist assistant as the physical therapy paraprofessional.

As personnel shortages and opportunities for physical therapist assistants continue, the need for a higher level of training will be important and essential. Evaluation skills used for gait training, (eg, when instructing in use of crutches for a patient with an ankle strain or sprain) will be a necessary skill for the assistant. Currently, if a physical therapist is not available for the gait training of such a patient, the task often is delegated to the emergency service nurse who may have had no training at all in that area. Assistants also may be aware of the need for further evaluation by a physical therapist, direct access laws could refer the patient. Other procedures that could be performed by the assistant may include: the application of transcutaneous electrical nerve stimulation, and instruction of the patient; measurement of range of motor and treatment, and evaluation of a wound and treatment. After initial findings are made, the physical therapist would determine further care to be given. The possibilities are endless and exciting. The abilities of physical therapist assistants are the key, and astute business persons will benefit from using creativity when working with administration and staff.

Conclusion

I believe that the members of the APTA will continue to have dialogue over the next five years that will be intriguing and thought-provoking. Practice issues of encroachment, direct access, rural practice settings and trends in health care will present new opportunities for assistants.

Controversy will continue to be associated with the physical therapist-physical therapist assistant relationship as physical therapist assistants become increasingly important in the delivery of physical therapy services.

The realization that fragmentation of the physical therapy profession could occur from a division between the classes of members of the Association over these controversial issues should make all members decide to become proactive and work together. Physical therapist assistants, in general, believe in a united, participatory existence with physical therapists in efforts to meet the challenges that face the profession in the future.

References
1. White BC: Physical therapy assistants: Implications for the Future Phys Ther 50:674-679, 1970.
2. Rutan FM: Implications of assistant-training programs for physical therapy: On licensure. Phys Ther 48:999-1002, 1968.

3. Committee on Supportive Personnel prepares Curriculum Guidelines for Physical Therapist Assistant Programs. Phys Ther 50:535-541, 1970.

4. Committee on Supportive Personnel prepares Guidelines for Physical Therapy Assistant Programs. Phys Ther 50:1355-1359, 1970.

5. Organizational Structure Task Force report: Scenario A1, A2, B1, B2. Progress Report of the American Physical Therapy Association 17 (1), 1988.

6. McDaniel LV: Formal training for assistants to physical therapists Phys Ther 42:562-565, 1962.

7. Killen MB: Supportive personnel in physical therapy. Phys Ther 47:483-490, 1967.

8. Holmes TM: Supportive personnel and supervisory relationships. Phys Ther 50:1165-1171, 1970.

9. Affiliate Special Interest Group Rules and Regulations. Alexandria, VA, American Physical Therapy Association, 1983 and 1987.

10. Evaluation of the American Physical Therapy Association: American Society of Association Executives. Alexandria, VA, American Physical Therapy Association, 1987.

11. Gray, JM: Function of Nonprofessional Physical Therapy Personnel. Phys Ther 44:103-109, 1964.

CHAPTER 6

Clinical Education: Forces for Change

Jane S. Mathews, MPH, PT

The forces for change in the clinical education for future physical therapy students come from a myriad of factors, including the relatively recent requirement for a postbaccalaureate degree. We, as physical therapists, must understand which factors influence our clinical education, which elements need to be changed, and what the ramifications are of some of our Association's actions. The purposes of this chapter relate to may personal perspectives about some of these forces for change; these opinions do not represent the official stance of the American Physical Therapy Association. Within the context of considerations about the impact of the postbaccalaureate degree education on the clinical education for future physical therapy students, I will discuss:

1. major contemporary trends and issues in the United States health care system and in the physical therapy professions
2. forces within physical therapy clinical and academic environments that also have implications for change in our clinical education modes
3. some courses of action I believe physical therapists may wish to consider when identifying and implementing desirable changes.

Background

As a basis for my perspectives, I need to qualify several issues. First, I believe that the indications for restructuring our clinical education modes were evident long before the APTA House of Delegates (HOD) enacted RC 14-79, which required postbaccalaureate degree education or physical therapists. This view is supported by findings reported as early as 1960 in a study by Dr. Catherine Worthingham that was on physical therapy education and practice. Additional evidence was reported in 1975 from the Section for Education's study conducted by Margaret Moore and associates that was on clinical education and in 1980 from a follow-up study by Dr. Jean Barr that was on clinical education standards. Unfortunately, many of the findings and recommendations contained in those reports were largely ignored.

Additionally, I believe that physical therapists need to remind themselves that the assumptions that underlie the profession's current mode(s) of clinical education may have questionable validity. This is not to say that the existing modes have failed to serve the profession well, because they have, as evidenced by all the competent educators and practitioners today. The assumptions, however, are in question because they were developed at a time when professional practice was very different. In my generation, for example, clinical education exposure in a few (ie, two or three) delivery settings made sense mainly because hospitals and rehabilitation centers were the major practice environments. With the expansion in physical therapists roles, functions, and practice settings over the past two decades and with the increased role emphasis on primary and secondary prevention, those original assumptions are elusive at best and no longer valid at worst.

Finally, I do not believe it is clear about what types of change are needed for our clinical education. Our current clinical education model must have been and must be effective in view of the performance of graduates in the health care marketplace. On the other hand, the physical therapists with whom I talk (ie, students, clinical faculty members, educators, practitioners) seem to sense that changes are needed. Students, for example, seem to think they have insufficient time allocated to clinical education experiences in their programs, clinical faculty members often state that they do not have enough time with students and that students come to them with less than adequate levels of competence for particular experiences, academic faculty members are frustrated because there is too little time allocated in a professional program because both the academic and clinical components seem to be "too short."

With these concerns and unanswered questions in mind, I will make recommendations for change and for what physical therapists should be aiming at in clinical education and in professional practice. As Henry David Thoreau said, "In the long run, men/women hit only what they aim at. Therefore, though they should fail immediately, they had better aim at something high."

Context of Decision-Making

The context within which the current decisions are being made about future clinical education has a strong influence on the factors considered and the potential for the final outcome. Three major areas of concern for physical therapists are the contemporary practices in the health care system, the current state of affairs in the physical therapy clinical and academic environments that call for change.

Current issues and trends in these areas are summarized in the following sections. The lists presented review the factors I consider having major influences on physical therapy decision making.

United States Health Care System

1. Cost containment is emphasized. The concept of cost containment is not new; it has been a part of the health care system since the late 1960s. The new aspect is the acknowledgment that with the immense and uncontrolled Federal budgetary deficit, societal and health care resources are finite. The heyday of expenditures is over for health care research, capital construction, payment for ever-expanding service provision, and subsidies to support the education of health personnel. The clear focus is on containing costs and spending.

The prospective payment systems (ie, Diagnostic Related Groups) initiated in hospitals for patients financed under the Medicare program merely are the tip of the iceberg in curtailing costs. Plans are underway to extend this system, in whatever refined form it eventually may emerge, to all other types of delivery environments and client populations. In effect, arguments of "high quality care" are not the issue; the reality orientation is "adequacy of care," which is not necessarily synonymous with high quality.

2. Increased requirements are emphasized for the justification and substantiation of the cost-effectiveness and essentialness of service interventions by type of provider. This refers not only to governmental third-party payers but also to the commercial and not-for-profit third parties such as Blue Cross and Blue Shield.

Physical therapists have long been vulnerable in their inabilities to demonstrate direct, cause-effect relationships between their therapeutic interventions and the outcomes in relation to their clients' problems. As providers, physical therapists may know intuitively that their interventions "work" in terms of obtaining functional outcomes for clients, but in many arenas they still lack the data to make those claims clear to third-party payers. I believe physical therapists still are being hurt from the results of the 1982 study by the General Accounting Office of the Federal government that indicated 32% of the physical therapy services rendered under the Medicare program constituted unnecessary care or over-utilization. Although less than desirable methodology can be said to have been used in that study, the data tend to be overwhelming, particularly in the examples given.

3. Procompetition is an increasingly valued concept. In relation to identifying the most cost-effective service interventions, health care providers (including physical therapists) are competing for the health care dollar. Therapists can complain to no avail about "infringements" on their turf because if another type of provider demonstrates a more cost-effective program for obtaining the desired functional outcomes for clients, the physical therapists' interventions traditionally considered to be theirs may become part of their history. Physical therapists, of course, can continue to argue that they have the better educational preparation, but I suspect that argument will fall on deaf ears because the outcomes or results of treatment will be a critical variable for the fiscal decision makers.

4. Primary and secondary prevention in health care has increased emphasis as compared with tertiary prevention in disability limitation and rehabilitation. Although tertiary prevention has been the role perceived as the major

focus of physical therapists, during the past decade they increasingly have become aware of and involved in wellness and health promotion activities. As an example, "early case-finding" and "screening for early intervention" are terms now found frequently in their vocabulary. Yet, primary and secondary prevention must become the most critical components the physical therapists' professional role and function.

5. Resources for the health care system are being directed increasingly to noninstitutional service settings (eg, various forms of ambulatory and out-of-hospital care). The American Hospital Association now seems to conceive the hospital as a "multiunit" corporation, with the in-patient unit being only one small (and perhaps most expensive to operate) facet of the total operation. For financial survival, many hospitals are attempting to develop, as a part of the multiunit corporation, a variety of out patient clinics and services. Some of these setups require physical therapists' involvement such as in sports injury or back screening clinics. Many of these setups, however, are developed as profit-sharing relationships with physicians and not the physical therapists who provide the bulk of the services. The physical therapists who work in these situations report that they often are reimbursed on a prorated (salary based) basis for providing such services above and beyond the regular work hours of their departments but are not offered the opportunity for profit-sharing participation.

6. The characterization of the health care system now is "decentralized decision-making." In terms of resource allocation decisions and programming, the activities now are at the state and local levels. That system differs from the one in the 1960s and 1970s when most of the activities occurred at the Federal government level in the Senate and House of Representatives. Physical therapists need to be cognizant of that change and be willing to invest effort and financing in their state legislatures for those proposed actions that would facilitate the most appropriate use of their services.

7. Awareness and sophistication of the health care consumer is increasing regarding self-responsibility for health behaviors. This change definitely is a positive factor in behalf of physical therapy, but therapists must develop better skills in cultivating their consumer support constituencies. Certainly, the lobbying of physical therapists and their lobbying representatives is crucial.

I suspect, however, that the lobbying of organized client constituents such as parents of children with neurodevelopmental problems or citizens in all age groups who personally have benefitted from physical therapy services would have a far greater impact on legislators at all levels than the input from the professionals who have an obvious self-interest.

8. Self-perceptions of professional roles and functions by physical therapists have far more sophisticated dimensions than the perceptions of these roles and functions by external groups in the health care system and in society. Physical therapists still are perceived largely as technicians who do nothing more than follow the specific orders of physicians. The APTA and the Section on Private Practice of the APTA have embarked on a major effort to modify that public image. My impression, however, is that the major responsibility rests with individual physical therapists and their behaviors in

their practice environments. What they as individuals do and how they behave will reflect on the profession as a whole. If therapists do not, cannot, or will not be prepared to substantiate their patient care decision-making, delineate their reasons for a particular treatment plan, or confront physicians and others on matters regarding the best interests of their patients, then they will have to be satisfied with a technician role. If they are not willing to exercise the accountability that is concomitant with professional responsibility, then the technician image will continue to be projected. If we, as physical therapists, prefer to be treated as health care professionals --and I believe most of us want to achieve that goal --then our behaviors must reflect those of professionals who are willing to be accountable, to substantiate decisions, and to take risks in behalf of the best interests of their clients.

Physical Therapy Profession

1. Legislative changes now allow physical therapy practice without referral. At the time of this writing, some twenty-one states have achieved legislative changes in their practice acts that now allow both evaluation and treatment without referral. One frequently asked question about these changes as they evolved and how it relates to the goal for postbaccalaureate degree education, is, "Does this mean that we will have to change our professional education programs in order to insure that graduates are prepared to function effectively in an independent mode of practice?"

I find this to be a rhetorical question. In fact, regardless of the substance of state practice acts, practice without referral became an issue in the HOD of the APTA because members in certain practice environments already were having to function in independent decision-making modes.

Personally, I am not convinced that our preparatory professional education has to change markedly because of the changes in practice legislation. My observation has been that for many years the education of physical therapists has provided the ability to make professional judgments at a level not permitted by the environments in which they function. In effect, I have no concerns about the capability of physical therapists as currently educated to function in an independent-practice-without-referral mode.

On the other hand, given the trend for independent practice, I believe changes can be made in the professional education programs that can enhance the decision-making, judgment, and practice of physical therapy graduates. I think that the terminal clinical competencies noted in the accreditation requirements merely need expansion. For example, many if not most physical therapy educational programs need more emphasis in primary and secondary prevention, pharmacology, business and management, and referral system capabilities. Because of the changes in the health care market-place, I also suspect that students need to have a higher level of mastery of some of these competence areas when they first enter the clinical education environment.

In sum, I would suggest that physical therapists have for some time been "over-educated" for the roles and functions that the health care marketplace allows them to demonstrate. This inequality should not be perceived as a negative factor, however, but should serve as a basis for making progress in resolving current practice issues and in meeting demands for demonstrating professional care.

2. A trend is developing toward specialization within physical therapy. During the past few years, much progress has been made in the process of developing formal board certification procedures to recognize specialization (advance competence) in the following areas of practice: cardiopulmonary care, pediatrics, orthopedics, sports physical therapy, neurology, and clinical electrophysiology. This movement started long before the postbaccalaureate degree issue and may or may not be associated with the latter. Specialization was inevitable as the body of knowledge and technology expanded in an exponential manner during the past two decades.

Confusion exists regarding the relationship of specialization and the postbaccalaureate degree goal. The latter is a first professional degree in a program designed to prepare generalists for practice, which is in accord with most published philosophy. Academicians apparently tend to think that a first professional degree program should provide the student with a broad-based practice foundation and that any type of specialization per se should derive from later experience.

From my personal perspective, I think it would be difficult to prepare a specialist in a first (or entry-level) professional degree program. The goal of such programs at entry level is to provide a foundation; few, if any, students matriculating in such preparational programs have the background to identify immediately a specialization tract. This goal serves to distinguish the entry-level postbaccalaureate degree programs from the postprofessional or postservice graduate degree programs that are designed for those individuals who are already credentialed and have experience in physical therapy.

3. Practice modes and settings are changing. The APTA membership survey data for 1978 and 1982-1984 indicated a decreasing proportion (47% down to 42%) of respondents employed in hospital settings. Although this percentage of decrease seems small, over a four to five year period it suggests a major trend. Concomitantly, those in personnel agencies and those making direct recruitment efforts from hospitals indicate increasing difficulty in attracting even new graduates to hospital settings.

No reports provide data explaining the trend, but from my experience and exit surveys of graduates from two institutions I theorize the following:

1. when seeking first employment positions, students tend to value available mentorship, continuing professional development opportunities, and stability in department staff;

2. clinical education experiences in hospital settings tend to have more of a negative than a positive effect on students in relation to their seeking positions after graduation;

3. private practice corporations tend to offer more scholarship and recruitment incentives than do hospital settings;

4. new graduates tend to identify private practice corporate settings that provide the mentorship, a broad array of clients and settings, and more professional development incentives than provided by hospitals. All this is not to suggest that hospital settings necessarily are a negative

environment for new physical therapy graduates; however, it does suggest that new graduates are less likely to find the hospital setting the most desirable setting, in accordance with their personal values and priorities, for their first employment experience after completing their preparation programs.

4. Physician-owned physical therapy services have developed. The concern inherent in this issue is the potential exploitation of physical therapy clients, the physical therapy profession, and the individual physical therapists who may find themselves in exploitative environments. Physician-owned services are a major concern because events in the health care marketplace are providing the incentive for physicians to develop such services for profit-making motives. First, this country has entered a phase where an oversupply of physicians exist, especially in some medical specialties. Second, study findings indicate that under conditions of increased competition, physicians' fees do not decrease; reports show that fees increase to maintain the standard of previous income. Third, physical therapy services provide one of the best income-generating sources for private practice environments.

If the major concern is the potential exploitation of the client and the profession (eg, referral for services not truly needed), then physician-owned services should not be the only target of concern. There is a long history of the physical therapy profession in hospitals being exploited over time, and there even are instances of clients and physical therapists in physical therapy-owned private privates being exploited. If exploitation is the issue, then, in social conscience, all environments or situations must be addressed in which exploitation is a potential.

Nonetheless, remember that the professional organization, the APTA, has no control to dictate the environments in which physical therapists choose to practice. If physical therapists choose to practice in physician-owned services or other settings that potentially exploit the client or the profession, those are their options. Of the reasons for working in those situations, no data has been reported. It has been suggested that new graduates appear to be recruited easily for employment in physician-owned services because they tend to be in debt when they leave school and the starting salaries offered by physicians are higher than those available in other settings. Another vulnerable group appears to be female physical therapists reentering the work force having been out of practice for a number of years for family reasons; physician-owned services have flexibility regarding work hours.

Academic and Clinical Settings

1. Academic institutions, both public and private, are struggling for financial viability. Higher education institutions are experiencing the same financial survival struggles as are hospitals and other health care delivery settings. In many situations, the institutions' struggles have been longer (since the early 1970s) and more difficult. To deal with the inflationary economy, most higher education institutions delayed capital repair and other activities during the 1970s if it required major investment. Those activities included adjustments in faculty salaries, which fell way behind the gap in the rest of the

economy, and improvements in physical environments, which included space, repairs, and expansion. Those who question the reality of the struggle for financial survival for those institutions should note the increased emphasis in recent years on recruitment and the sophisticated marketing devices used to entice larger student enrollments, particularly in undergraduate programs.

2. Pressure has increased for maintaining or increasing enrollments in physical therapy programs. Physical therapy applicant pools have been among the best both qualitatively and quantitatively. Therefore, when other applicant or enrollment pools declined, increased pressure was placed on physical therapy and other viable programs. Unfortunately, increased resources, such as faculty positions, space, and equipment, have not necessarily been coexistent with increased enrollment pressures.

3. Faculty members are pressured for productivity. While the increased enrollment and matriculation demands are imposed on physical therapy faculty, they simultaneously are having to meet the traditional demands for academic credibility and survival within their institutions. For all intents and purposes, this means research and scholarly productivity essential for survival through the promotion and tenure process. Nothing is dysfunctional about that requirement provided that the physical therapy faculty have adequate opportunities related to time and resources to pursue those activities as part of the total academic professional role. Unfortunately, in many environments the physical therapy faculty are engaged primarily in teaching activities, either through individual orientation or institutional pressure. This activity bodes well for the student but does not bode well for the individual faculty member's productivity and survival. Professional academicians, physical therapists and otherwise, have a three-legged stool of responsibility that includes teaching, service-practice, and research. The fact remains that research and productivity in the scholarly sense (publication) remains one of the most valued criteria for promotion and tenure.

4. Educational philosophy or rationale of programs are not delineated clearly. Many academicians find themselves in settings where they automatically become "apprentices" to what they experienced as students. The philosophy and rationale of the program in which they are involved is developed but largely ignored because they are doomed, by the nature of the situation, to do only what they personally have experienced or what they know. The conscious and deliberate development of learning experiences within the context of a well-established program philosophy and rationale takes a highly mature and integrated faculty collective. Few physical therapy faculties have the time and inclination to develop that type of collective phiolosophical orientation.

5. Educational programs are costly to students. There is no doubt that physical therapy education is expensive whether at the baccalaureate, master's, or certificate level; therefore, many students graduate from existing programs deeply in debt from loans. Also, other types of costs are incurred. Both financial and social sacrifices are made in the students' lives and family situations to pursue physical therapy education. One such cost relates to the stress, program demands, and concentration required of physical therapy

students as they have to forego the social development opportunities afforded to other undergraduate and graduate students. From my experience, I believe that entry-level postbaccalaureate degree students have resolved this issue more functionally than baccalaureate degree majors. Perhaps I note this difference because the former have more life experiences as a basis for formulating physical therapy career decisions. The question, however, is whether a human service professional needs opportunities for social and intellectual development as well as professional education input.

6. Total academic faculty is not involved in clinical education. In many physical therapy education settings, the clinical education planning, involvement, and evaluation is left to the Academic Coordinator of Clinical Education. In one sense, that plan is understandable, but it raises other types of questions and issues. Should all the faculty be involved in such activities as clinical site visits, planning, and evaluations as a means of ensuring sufficient and relevant feedback "loops" between those in clinical practice and academic instruction? Current practice is changing so rapidly that some contact with a contemporary clinical environment seems essential for all physical therapy faculty, particularly those responsible for clinically oriented instruction. Yet, for reasons identified earlier, it frequently is not time efficient for all faculty members to have an active role in clinical site visits or other aspects of clinical education.

7. Pressures for academicians to specialize are increasing. The physical therapy faculty are challenged to keep up with the specialization that has occurred in the marketplace. On the one hand, all faculty members desire to be contemporary in their instruction to students. On the other hand, it is very difficult to differentiate that which is entry-level competence from that which is advanced competence. All too frequently, this decision rests with the individual faculty member's expertise and personal view of practice environments, which may or may not be contemporary or accurate. In some respects, how much of what is offered to students in any program is a direct function of expertise of the total faculty mix. Variability in total faculty strengths and expertise, therefore, may account for the unevenness or variability in the products of the entry-level programs.

8. Clinical settings may develop problems because of prospective reimbursement. To date, all the ramifications of the use of Diagnostic Related Groups for reimbursement have not been clear, but there are a number of definite implications. Regarding clinical education, a beginning picture is one of difficulty in the clinical environment in having time to invest in student supervision. At best this may mean fewer students accepted for placement; at worst this may mean discontinuance of clinical education opportunities for students.

Some clinical educators already have indicated an awareness of the loss of patients' extended availability for teaching purposes. Others have stated that initial encounters with patients may be the only opportunities students have for clinical learning. Considering the nuturing tradition that physical therapy faculty have with students, this could present problems.

9. Reward systems are needed for physical therapy clinical faculty. Historically, physical therapy clinical faculty have received few, if any, tangible

rewards for the time and effort they provide in behalf of student learning experiences. Few academic programs are in the financial position of offering direct financial reimbursement. Most, if not all, offer "cash in kind" options such as tuition credit vouchers, library services, or official faculty appointments. The issue seems to relate basically to recognition of clinical faculty efforts as an essential and integral part of any professional education program. Remember, however, that what is perceived to constitute appropriate recognition on the part of therapists may not coincide with the perceptions of appropriate recognition on the part of the institutions when considering the time and effort invested.

10. Clinical faculty need involvement in academic planning. Interestingly, most physical therapy academicians and clinical faculty express that such joint involvement would be of value; however, involvement seldom occurs to the extent desirable, particularly because all those involved cannot attend regular meetings together. Nonetheless, mechanisms can be found to foster and facilitate clinical faculty involvement through various department committees, advisory councils, and special task forces or through general elective representation of clinical faculty. This involvement is not easy and requires a strong value commitment on the part of the academic program director and full-time academic faculty to find ways to obtain the clinical faculty involvement.

11. The purpose of clinical education and the role of clinical faculty are misunderstood. Many clinical faculty, academicians, and students have unrealistic expectations of the clinical education experience and the role of clinical faculty. Sometimes, the clinical faculty perceive that they must be all things to all people, have the answers to all questions posed by students, and take full responsibility for the total development of their students. Likewise, students often have unrealistic expectations of their clinical supervisors by failing to remember that physical therapy now is diverse and that not all supervisors have experience in all areas of physical therapy. Academicians who have had to deal with time constraints in the didactic curriculum entertain the fantasy that the clinical education experience will fill in all the missing pieces and bring it all together for the students.

The responsibility for the success of the clinical education experience by no means rests fully with the clinical faculty. It is shared responsibility among and between the student, the academic program, and the clinical facility; it is integrally related to the needs of the student, the goals of the program, and the resources available in the clinical environment.

I suspect that physical therapy clinical faculty perceive a special burden because research in physical therapy and in other professions indicates that clinicians are the primary role models for students. Being a primary role model does not necessarily mean that a clinician can be made totally responsible or made to take the blame for what does or does not happen with a student.

The success of an individual student's clinical education experience is related strongly to planning, timing, the match between the student's needs and goals and the experiences available in the facility, and the validity of expectations of all parties concerned. Again, the responsibility is shared among and between the student, the academic program, and the clinical facility; each party involved must assume an equal proportion of that responsibility.

Proposed Courses of Action

The prevailing notion is evident that the clinical education component of physical therapy must change, but the nature and extent of those changes are subject to controversy. Given the forces and factors identified thus far, I will discuss predominant proposals and their possible validity and then make a few alternative proposals.

1. Increase the length of time directed to clinical education in the entry-level curricula. From the students' perspective, this notion appears to be justified; it is the most frequently mentioned variable in regard to changing our current clinical education mode and certainly merits consideration.

Many students have indicated to me that even at the end of eight-week clinical education assignments they are just beginning to understand the subculture and political nuances of the setting and just becoming able to organize and plan client-care programs. Likewise, clinical employers of new graduates tell me that it takes an average of six to nine months before a new graduate becomes adept in terms of time and work load organization and productivity. Many academicians have stated that extended time in clinical environments is essential for students to be able to integrate all the theory with practice and translate it into organized professional performance.

The rationales just stated all seem to have merit. I, however, submit that merely extending the length of the clinical education requirement is not solution in and of itself. Consider the following alternatives.

Alternative proposal: First, obtain a clear delineation of the type of competence and level of mastery necessary for effective physical therapy practice in the contemporary and anticipated future practice environments. Then, use that information as a basis for identifying the nature and extent of clinical and academic experiences necessary to develop a student to that point.

Alternative proposal: Given the clear delineation of competence and level of mastery, develop some valid and reliable entry-level performance standards as a basis for assessing the students' achievements of the desired behaviors.

At present, this assessment is a judgment left solely to the clinical faculty in relation to a particular environment. At times, however, the final assessment outcome is reversed by the academic faculty. I believe the physical therapy profession has evolved to the point of having the methods and capability of developing a more objective set of performance criteria that all students must meet prior to being judged competent to enter practice.

Another consideration is that few programs have been able to accommodate those students who develop desired levels of competence more rapidly than other students. It seems the programs more easily provide additional experiences for those students who may take longer to develop than to adjust to those students who take less time for whatever reason. Valid, reliable, and standardized performance criteria would allow the programs to accommodate both types of needs while being more accountable to the clinical environments that employ new graduates.

2. Establish loops of interactive accountability between the academic settings and the clinical settings. This proposal is difficult to argue with; however, the issue relates to how this could be accomplished. Historically, physical therapists have prided themselves that their clinical education has been designed consciously as planned learning experiences and that their students, therefore, have been nurtured zealously.

Alternative proposal: Change the traditional philosophy so that the total loop (ie, academic and clinical learning experiences) becomes a process of mutual audit in relation to the practice competence developed.

At present, only partial loops exist, with most of the auditing targeted to clinical education settings. My suggestion is to devise ways to complete this loop to ensure continuing input to the relevancy of content and processes taught in the academic component of the professional curriculum. This change opposes the "town and gown" concept, which I think has endured long enough. Because clinicians and academicians are functioning in very different environments and encounter differing forces, these differences must be acknowledged so that a better understanding can be developed of each others' environments and the programs for students can benefit.

3. Prepare students for practice without referral. Proponents of this view often lack specificity when questioned. I believe this consideration is needed because, as I have stated before, physical therapy educational programs have for some time been preparing students for a level of judgmental decision making not always permitted in their practice environments.

Alternative proposal: Confront the reality of contemporary practice environments and construct the types of academic and clinical learning experiences that will facilitate the development of clinical reasoning and problem-solving skills.

Perhaps more attention should be given to how the learning experiences are constructed rather than to what content is included. If the nature of the learning experiences in both environments relates to "do as I do or do as I say," then the obedience-to-authority-figure syndrome is perpetuated.

This problem is further perpetuated by a pedagogical mode that emphasizes undirectional lectures and regurgitation of specifics rather than opportunities to test concepts and discuss, analyze, apply, and present comparative rationales and substantiation.

4. Provide clinical education experiences in a variety of health delivery settings. I question whether the key is the setting or if it is the needs of the client population and the role and function of the physical therapist in relation to those needs. Physical therapists, for example, are most likely to encounter clients with cerebrovascular accidents in both hospital and home care settings; however, the nature of the problems presented by the clients and the roles and functions of physical therapists vary in each of the settings.

Alternative proposal: Develop clinical education consortiums in defined geographic areas and design them around a variety of client needs and problems rather than the settings per se. This means a student might go to a particular geographic area, remain in one living location, and rotate through a variety of service experiences and client populations. A student with particular development needs potentially could spend longer periods of time in the setting with the client population most suitable to the development of the needed performance behaviors. As an additional consideration, conceptualize clinical education within the context of the personal health service spectrum by incorporating activities related to primary, secondary, and tertiary prevention (eg, health promotion and specific protection, case finding and early intervention, and traditional disability limitation and rehabilitation activities).

5. Provide extended internship or residency opportunities for physical therapists after completion of basic professional education requirements. Experimentation with the extended internship at the University of Southern California many years ago tends to support this notion. On the other hand, this consideration may relate to a more basic issue than that indicated by the proposed course of action.

Alternative proposal: Develop a consciously planned career structure in physical therapy that begins with the earliest years of higher education and extends to preparation for formal board certification in a specialty area.

Physical therapists as professionals tend to be quick to reject anything that suggests a medical model. There are career structuring aspects of the medical model, however, that warrant attention and consideration. In the present physical therapy education scheme (including physical therapy aides trained on the job, two-year associate degree physical therapist assistants, the existing three types of entry-level professional programs, and the postprofessional education programs), little exists to suggest any conscious planning for articulation with long-run career development in mind. From a personal perspective, it makes no sense to make major decisions about entry-level professional programs without simultaneously identifying the potential impact on or changes needed in physical therapist assistant programs and postprofessional graduate programs. To be concerned with these aspects requires attention to the planning of a career structure that so far has not been addressed by the profession or its professional organization.

Additionally, even in developing recognized speciality areas, the physical therapy profession has ignored the needs of the individual who opts to become an expert "generalist" in physical therapy. This component would be essential to consider in career structure development.

Summary

The major forces that will influence the development of clinical education in the physical therapy profession come from multiple factors both internal and external to the official organization. To enhance decision making for the clinical education of future physical therapists, it is essential to develop an awareness of the relevant issues and trends within the context of the contemporary health care system, the physical therapy profession in general, and the physical therapy clinical and academic settings. This awareness should include controversial points of view from the standpoint of legislation, physicians' practices, hospital administration, physical therapy clinical and academic faculty, students, new graduates, practitioners, and clinical specialists. The ramifications of any decisions regarding all of these elements must be considered before future changes are instituted. Prevailing proposals for change must be evaluated carefully for validity, and alternative choices must be considered in light of new information.

same delivery vehicle could offer services and receive reimbursement from other payers. In retrospect, it would appear that this cost reimbursement system established by Medicare succeeded in encouraging the demonstration of care related costs. More costs were incurred when higher salaries were paid, more programs developed, and more treatment was given. These practices, while supporting cost allowances on the Medicare cost report, also greatly increased payments made to health care providers by other payment sources. Physical therapists benefited from the climate that promoted program development within facilities at a time when they were developing their unique professional skills and knowledge toward an expanded array of patient diagnoses and practice settings. Unfortunately, the profession was represented among those that exploited the system in the respect that overutilization and delivery of unnecessary or incomplete services was practiced.

By the late 1970s and the early 1980s, reaction to burgeoning health costs was well established and became evident in both public and private sectors. As changes in health care were occurring, public policy and opinion also were shifting. Issues of community response to health and human needs were being downplayed in favor of messages of self-sufficiency and the need for public "belt tightening." In the private sector, employers that purchased health care coverage for their employees were not accepting routine premium increases and the insurance industry saw a development of a wide array of health care benefit products that created a competitive atmosphere in that industry. In the public sector, increase in regulations was the initial response to calls for restraint. Outside providers of physical therapy attempted a rational, logical approach to the proposed salary equivalence regulations, and they were somewhat surprised with the uncompromising responses and zeal in mission that they perceived was present on the part of Health Care Financing Administration (HCFA) officials. Outside suppliers of physical therapy were those who provided service to a Medicare agency (eg, hospital, home health agency) on a fee for service rather than a salaried basis. The salary equivalence laws established limits on the costs that could be attributed to those professional fees. In addition, medical review of care provided resulted in increased incidence of retroactive denial of payment for services rendered. Derivations of these methods of cost containment were adopted by other third party payers, and many of those payers made arrangements for medical review of the services they provided. A new component of the reimbursement industry developed: benefits "management" companies that contracted with employers or insurance companies to reduce health care costs through strict claims review. It was not unusual for those contracts to be based on a guaranteed benefits reduction.

An alternative response to increased costs and overutilization of services has been the emergence of prepaid health plans and the prospective payment system that HCFA has established for hospital care of Medicare patients. Both approaches are similar in the respect that responsibility for variances from projected costs are shifted to the health care provider.

It is striking that much of the policy and practice relevant to the reimbursement of health care has been a result of reaction to public need or health care practice. Now that reimbursement policy is making an impact on health care

CHAPTER 7

Issues and Trends in Reimbursement

Mary R. Daulong, BS, PT
Mari F. Nye, BS, PT

Issues and Trends in Health Care Reimbursement

For nearly the first half of the 1900s, the delivery of health care was simplistic, clinically and administratively, and its financing was a personal matter between the provider and the patient. After World War II and into the early 1960s, the health care industry enjoyed an uncontested growth explosion. That growth was directed to delivering a rapidly expanding array of services to a public that was developing a consciousness that the best in health care was an entitlement of the American way of life. Public policy championed human services with broad legislative programs, exemplified in the health care arena by the Medicare program, established in 1965. Employers offered health care insurance as a fringe benefit, and full comprehensive coverage packages were seen as an asset of value in recruiting and labor relations. During this period of growth, professional activity in the physical therapy profession was directed to identifying its role in health care and to advocating the inclusion of physical therapy services in the community of providers and in the reimbursement manuals in the "covered services" section.

With the inception of Medicare in 1965, providing health care and financing health care became big business. Medicare was designed to be a cost reimbursement program, with the intention that public funds should not be used to contribute to profit for health care providers. Health care providers learned that Medicare reimbursement for demonstrated costs could finance a vehicle for service delivery that could be used to generate profit when that practice trends, it is essential that physical therapists who wish to deliver high quality professional care as well as survive in the current environment make commitments to a knowledge of reimbursement terminology and third party practices.

It is worthwhile to examine some general trends in the administration practices of reimbursement sources. Major payers have come "on line" and use computer technology to improve the efficiency of their own organizations. The data collection and analysis available through this technology likely are giving the third-party-payer industry a more generalized picture of the physical therapy profession's utilization patterns than they had previously. In addition, the desire to use computer technology for claims review process requires a set of presumptions about the nature of intervention that is appropriate in a given claims situation. In this type of environment, consideration of claims on an individual basis becomes quite difficult.

At the very least, these developments point to a need for establishing uniform and consistent reference terminology. Aside from ethical infractions, particularly utilization abuses, physical therapists discredit themselves most with third party payers when they fail to be uniform and consistent in referring to physical therapy services.

Presuming that therapists can develop the language that will clarify for third party payers who therapists are and what they do, they need to understand who the reimbursement sources are and how they pay.

The term third party payer is a generic expression covering three entities: private insurance companies, government health programs with claims payment agents, independent health plans.

Pursuing reimbursement or claims payment can be difficult if a person does not know which classification a payer fits into because regulations and reimbursement characteristics vary from entity to entity.

Private Health Insurance Company Classifications

In the private health insurance industry within the United States, there are three types of firms: commercial stock companies, mutual companies, and nonprofit insurance plans. Important organizational differences exist among these insurers. The primary variances are as follows:

The *stock companies* (such as Aetna, Travelers, and Connecticut General) are private stockholder owned corporations and operate in the national marketplace.

The *mutual companies* (like Mutual of Omaha, Prudential, and Metropolitan Life) also deal in the national market and have private holders; however, they differ because the policyholders also are the owners.

Both stock and mutual companies are called commercial carriers, and they are subject to state insurance laws and state and federal taxation.

Nonprofit insurance plans (Blue Cross, Blue Shield, and Delta Dental) are granted exclusive franchises to geographical areas and to a particular line of insurance. These carriers are subject to stringent state regulations but are tax exempt because of their nonprofit status.

Private health insurance companies typically reimburse providers of physical therapy service on a fee for service basis. Fee for service payment can range from being fairly simple to relatively complex. Fee for service categories are billed charges; fixed fee schedules; payment based on usual, customary, and reasonable charges; and relative value schedules.

The traditional and most simple form of reimbursement under fee for service is *billed charges*. The provider independently sets his fees and bills the patient directly for them. Although this method is simple, it carries high risks of having a significant bad debt rate because the provider also is the collector of all payments.

Use of a *fixed fee schedule* is a favored method of the payer group because they have some control over prices; this system obviously is not preferred by the provider for the same reason. Although the fixed fee system can be administered very simply, it can be complicated easily by establishing fee schedules according to class of provider or location. Payments are made either directly to the patient (indemnifications) or directly to the provider (reimbursement). If the indemnification method is chosen, the patient is reimbursed within the fixed fee guidelines by the payer but billed by the provider at his fee for service. The payer's fixed fees generally are less than but never greater than the provider's fees. If direct reimbursement is chosen, there may be two options for the provider: assignment of benefits or non-assignment of benefits. If the provider has the option and chooses to accept an assignment, he then agrees to accept the fixed fees from the third party payer as payment in full, exclusive of coinsurance payments and deductibles. If there is a nonassignment option and the provider chooses it, he is reimbursed by the payer at the fixed rate, however, he is free to bill the payment for the outstanding amount. This procedure is called balanced billing. Many providers reject assignments because they question the payer's advertent or inadvertent control of fees. Additionally, depending on a state's regulation, balanced billing may not be used for services provided to Workers' Compensation beneficiaries.

With the fixed fee schedule under fire, a new but much more complicated method of payment was developed by Blue Shield. This new system was called *payment based on usual, customary and reasonable charges*, which is known as UCR within the insurance industry. This procedure involves collecting fee data for each participating provider and arranging that data into profiles. The UCR profiles and related procedures can be used singularly but generally are used in combination.

The first profile is the *usual fee* and it is defined as the median charge. (Actual practice, however, appears to obtain a mean rather a median.) This median charge is derived from a listing of actual fees charged by a provider for a specific service within a given period of time. Once all providers have established medians for comparable services, the medians are ranked in order from the lowest to the highest usual charge per provider, resulting in a second profile called *customary charges*. The percentile cap, above which the payer does not pay, is placed on this profile by most UCR payers; this cap generally varies from 75% to 95% of the customary charges. The percentile cap is a negative feature only for those providers with high usual charges.

When calculating *reasonable charges*, the payers reimburse at the lowest of actually billed fee, at the provider's own usual fee, or at the percentile cap on the customary charges.

What clearly is evident when examining the UCR payment scheme is that it is an administrative nightmare, with the primary burden on the payer. Because this system fosters long term fee control by providers, payers have been forced to reduce percentile caps or levy freezes on usual charges.

The *relative value schedule* (RVS) evolved as a result of the power struggle between provider and payer over fee, or price, control. The relative value schedule also is less cumbersome to administer and is implemented easily. The first step in implementing the RVS is to establish a monetary value for a unit. Next, each service is weighted and assigned units; a consideration of the provider's qualifications and skills as well as time involved is included when the unit assignment is made. Payment is made by calculating the number of units performed by the provider and multiplying that total by the predetermined monetary value. The RVS is less cumbersome than other payment methods discussed thus far and represents compromise between the reimbursement industry and the providers.

Government Health Insurance Classifications

The government health plans are represented by Medicare, Medicaid, the Federal Employees Health Benefits Plans, and the Civilian Health and Medical Program of the Uniformed Service (CHAMPUS). The federal government may administer its plans through use of a claims payment agent. A claims payment agent is a private contractor responsible for managing the payment process for specific government health plans. These claims payment agents have different titles, depending which program they are managing. They are called intermediaries when dealing with Part A Medicare, carriers when dealing with Part B Medicare, and fiscal agents when working with the state Medicaid programs.

The Medicare program administers and reimburses for services covered that have utilized methods specific to the classification of the service provider.

Prospective payment is being used currently for inpatient hospitalization and is being developed for other health care providers. Medicare pays the provider (hospital) a set amount, depending on the patient's admission diagnosis. That set amount is based on the number of hospital days that was determined to be associated with that diagnosis. If a patient is discharged in less than the projected days, the prospective payment amount may represent a revenue gain for the hospital; a stay that extends beyond the projected days or an admission that is considered inappropriate (not on the list of approved diagnoses) may represent a revenue loss for the hospital.

Cost reimbursement, a method used previously for services provided in the hospital, continues to be used for payment of other providers, including rehabilitation agencies, home health agencies, skilled nursing facilities, and certified outpatient rehabilitation facilities. Payment is made based on the costs that are demonstrated to be necessary to deliver those services. Payment may be received on an intermittent basis, based on a unit of delivery (eg, home health visit) in the course of a year; however, that year's costs and services are demonstrated retrospectively through a cost report, and a payee may be asked to refund funds should some of the costs be disallowed as unreasonable.

Independent practitioners who are providers of service to Medicare beneficiaries may be certified as Medicare providers. A *fee for service* payment method which is analogous to the usual, customary, and reasonable payment method, is used to determine payment and, in some cases, a maximum per calendar year per beneficiary per provider is set.

The Medicaid program, though a federal entitlement, is administered through state agencies and coverage and reimbursement methodology varies from state to state.

Independent Health Plans

Independent health plans are organized by groups such as consumer cooperatives, unions, and university medical groups. Health maintenance organizations and self-insurance plans also fall within this category. Enrollment in these types of plans, particularly the health maintenance organizations, is increasing at this time. The state regulations that apply to the health care plans differ from those that apply to private insurance companies and typically involve increased specification of the amount and types of services that will be offered to plan members.

Reimbursement for services provided to beneficiaries of these plans typically is a method of either fee for service or capitation. When a provider is reimbursed by the fee for service method, that fee usually is negotiated in advance for a specific term.

Capitation is a simple payment method. A fixed fee, prepaid by the provider, is actually based on comprehensive care over a specific period of time for a particular number of enrollees who have agreed to use the designated provider. Quality care and utilization issues arise when a potential for profit exists associated with nondelivery of care. Viewed in a positive light, the profit potential could be represented as an incentive for excellent preventive care.

Physical therapists may provide care for health plan members as an employee of the plan or an employee of one of the designated providers. Alternatively, physical therapists may be reimbursed on a fee for service or a capitation basis.

Summary

A description of the physical therapy profession's present disposition in light of the evolution of trends in reimbursement does point, it seems, to present needs.

1. Uniform terminology and reference language is needed to facilitate dialogue with reimbursement agents.
2. A distinct, positive identification with third party payers needs to be established that is supported by clinical research substantiating professional intervention as inseparable from functional outcome.

Beyond addressing current needs, we would advocate for physical therapists to assume responsibility as proactive participants in determining reimbursement practices and policies. Physical therapists have been discredited by practices of overutilization and misrepresentation. Therapists must respond to this discredit through unified aggressive action. Physical therapy must be synonymous with achievement of functional outcome. With efforts invested toward that level of accountability, the profession could expect to achieve validation and distinction. Reimbursement based on achievement of functional outcome would promote sound decision making by physical therapists and greater incentive by patients to assume a share of responsibility for their functional accomplishments. Excellence in practice would be reimbursed in kind. Physical therapists must be willing to address changes. The alternative is to continue to face the future of reimbursement as it relates to physical therapists being contented/discontented spectators and reactors as the development may dictate.

Selected Readings

Aetna and hospital group set health plan venture. Wall Street Journal, April 2, 1985.

Blue Cross bed system draws debate. Wall Street Journal, December 2, 1984.

California physical therapists in private practice form their own PPO seeking representation in marketplace. Hospitals, November 16, 1985.

Hickok RJ (ed): Physical Therapy Administration and Management, ed 2. Baltimore, MD, Williams and Wilkins, 1982.

Horting M: Reimbursement systems react to cause changes in health care delivery. Progress Report of the American Physical Therapy Association 15(9), 1986.

Insurers Change in Approach may threaten hospitals' margins. Modern Healthcare, February 1, 1985, p 49-52.

Major changes are predicted for group health coverage. Business Insurance, June 18, 1984, p 12.

Reducing health care costs with a preferred provider organization. Business, January 1985, p 22-26.

The preferred provider organization (PPO) offers hope for control of sky rocketing health care rates. Industry Week, September 19, 1983, p 19-20.

Waldholz M: Businesses are forming coalitions to curb rise in health care costs. Wall Street Journal, June 11, 1982p.

References

1. Rapoport J, Robertson RL, Stuart B: Understanding Health Economics. Rockville, MD, Aspen Publishers, Inc. 1982.

CHAPTER 8

Understanding and Influencing the Legislative Process

George G. Olsen, Esq.*

As physical therapists chart the future course of their profession, they will have to be prepared to navigate the uncertain and often turbulent waters of the Congressional legislative process. There looms on the horizon a plethora of issues that will mandate physical therapists to become more intimately involved in that process than ever before. The professional objectives of securing practice without referral and alleviating the abuses attendant to referral for profit situations will be achieved, at least in part, through federal legislation. Similarly, as the President and Congress work to restructure Medicare, Medicaid, veterans health programs, and other social services, physical therapists will be compelled to participate legislatively to ensure that their welfare, and the welfare of their patients, are protected adequately. Just as the enactment of the prospective payment system for inpatient hospital services demanded that physical therapists actively protect their interests, so too will the impending proposals to extend prospective payment to outpatient services and to move toward a capitated system of federal reimbursement for health care services. The private sector providers and suppliers of health care services and the consumers of such services (both individual and corporate) will be the source of significant and far-reaching legislation as they attempt to modify existing health care delivery systems or establish alternative delivery systems to suit their own needs. Physical therapists will need to play a role in these reforms as well.

---

*Mr. Olsen is a member of the law firm of Williams & Jensen, PC; which represents numerous health care associations and providers of health care. The firm was the general counsel to the American Physical Therapy Association for over 12 years.

In addition, the effectiveness of the American Physical Therapy Association (APTA) on legislative endeavors would be enhanced immeasurably if individual members of the Association became involved actively in the political and legislative processes. The design of this monograph is to explain why such participation is extremely important, describe legislative procedures in a fashion that laymen can understand, and suggest ways in which physical therapists can influence legislation.

> *No man's property or life is safe while the legislature is in session.* —
> Unknown New England Judge

During the heat of battle over health care legislation, one factor, albeit often the most important, frequently receives scant attention—the impact of the legislation on providers of services and the effect of legislation on the scope and quality of services available to patients. The burgeoning federal deficit has placed principle emphasis on the macroeconomic effect of legislation, that is, will it reduce or exacerbate the deficit or is it "budget neutral." Proposals that add to federal expenditures will face extremely rough sledding even though they may improve patient care substantially. Conversely, measures that may be inimical to quality care often will find acceptance because they help reduce the federal deficit.

The influence of the deficit on health care legislation was intensified by the passage of the Balanced Budget and Emergency Deficit Control Act. This law, commonly known as the Gramm-Rudman-Hollings Act, sets deficit reduction target amounts for each year over a five-year period, at the end of which the federal deficit will have been eliminated. If the target is not met in any given year, a sequestration order may be issued providing for across-the-board spending cuts sufficient to reduce the deficit to the target level. The effects of sequestration are so onerous that legislators will go to great lengths to avoid the imposition of such an order. As a result of the Gram-Rudman-Hollings Act and the rules that the Senate and House have adopted pursuant to it, legislation has become a zero-sum game. Simply put, the deficit reduction target acts as a bottom-line outcome and all legislation must be balanced and tailored to comply with that objective. Programs may be expanded only if others are cut back to compensate or if additional sources of revenue (eg, new or higher taxes) are found.

This zero-sum approach to legislation is revolutionary and places enormous burdens on participants in the legislative process. If physical therapists, for example, were to seek legislation requiring increased federal spending, an extremely strong showing that this legislation was necessary would have to be made to convince legislators that the physical therapy amendment should be adopted at the expense of funding for some other program. Similarly, physical therapists must be prepared to demonstrate that programs and benefits important to them or their patients should not be cut in order to fund some other interest's amendment.

> *War is much too serious a matter to be entrusted to the military.*
> —Georges Clemenceau

The protection of the interests of physical therapists is surely far too important to entrust to the beneficence of the United States Congress. Given the enormity of the federal deficit problem and the complexity of the statutory and regulatory devices that have been implemented to resolve it, however, one could query reasonably what individual physical therapists could do to ensure that the interests of the profession are guarded. The answer rests in two simple facts. First, physical therapists know more about their profession and the needs of their patients than any senator, congressman, or federal regulator. Physical therapists alone have the expertise and experience to develop the evidence to justify their legislative initiatives. Second, physical therapists have the constitutional right to support and vote for members of congress and other elected officials who share their views on health care issues. The zero-sum protocol currently permeating the legislative process demands that individual physical therapists utilize these inherent powers and rights to help its representatives in Washington, DC, to secure passage of beneficial legislation.

To a legislator, the importance, of the knowledge physical therapists have about their profession and patients cannot be overstated. Physical therapists, not legislators, have the training and hands-on experience to know what constitutes quality care. Physical therapists, not politicians, are in daily contact with aged, infirmed, and injured individuals, and, therefore understand well the physical, financial, and emotional aspects of their care. Only physical therapists can appreciate fully the microeconomic effect that legislation enacted by Congress will have on them and their patients.

The key to a successful legislative campaign, especially now that deficit considerations dominate the legislative process, is the willingness and ability of individual physical therapists to augment the efforts of the APTA by apprising their congressmen and senators of issues important to physical therapists and giving them the evidence that will lead them to support physical therapy proposals. To be effective grassroots lobbyists, physical therapists must understand the legislative process and know how to establish lines of communication with their elected representatives. It is to these issues, that this document now turns.

> *Don't let the public see either the making of sausages or of the law*
> —Otto von Bismarck

Despite Bismarck's admonition, a basic understanding of the legislative procedures of the US Congress is necessary for anyone who contemplates becoming involved in the legislative arena. What follows is a very simplified description of that process.

Introduction of Measure

Any member of the House or the Senate may introduce (ie, sponsor) legislation. It may be prepared by the member, his staff, a committee staff, a constituent, or other organization. There are four types of legislation. A "bill" is the proper form for any type of general public legislation and is the most common. Final action on a bill is the President's signature at which time it becomes public law. A "joint resolution" follows the same procedure as a bill, but the legislative purposes of such measures are usually incidental or unusual in nature (eg, extending a welcome to a foreign dignitary). A "concurrent resolution" is agreed to by both the House and the Senate, does not become public law, and is used to express principles and opinions of the two bodies. A resolution involves only one chamber and embraces subjects pertaining solely to the House or Senate as a body —(eg, a change in procedure).

At the adjournment of each two-year Congress, all bills that have not become law die and must be reintroduced in the next Congress in order to receive consideration. During the 99th Congress, nearly 8,000 measures were introduced in the House and 4,000 in the Senate. Most were not acted.

Referral to Committee

After introduction, each measure is referred to the congressional committee which has jurisdiction over the subject matter of the bill. The Senate and House have differing committee jurisdictions and names. For example, the Ways and Means Committee and the Energy and Commerce Committee have jurisdiction over health matters in the House, but the Committee on Finance has such jurisdiction in the Senate. A bill may be referred to a single committee or to two or more committees if there is joint or overlapping jurisdiction among several committees. Bills that have been jointly referred must be acted by each of the committees before the legislation may be brought to the floor for a vote. Split referral may occur when different parts of a bill fall within the subject matter jurisdiction of more than one committee. In such instances, each committee exercises jurisdiction over the portion that falls within its purview.

Committee Action

Committee action usually begins with one of the committee's subcommittees. A subcommittee may hold hearings on a given subject, and any bills dealing with that subject may be considered in such hearings. Persons interested in the legislation may submit written or oral testimony. Under normal circumstances, the executive branch agency which has responsibility for the subject area of the legislation will be asked to testify.

Following subcommittee hearings, the members and staff consider changes in proposed legislation based on information elicited during the hearings and obtained from various sources. This may be done informally or during a "markup" session of the subcommittee. After markup, the subcommittee may report the bill favorably or unfavorably to the full committee, with or without amendment, or suggest that it be "tabled."

The full committee then may conduct additional hearings or proceed directly to a markup session. For a bill to be reported out to the floor, a majority of the committee must vote in favor of it. After a markup session, a "committee report" is prepared that contains an explanation of the provisions of the measure; its cost; its inflationary impact; and supplementary, minority, or additional views of individual members of the full committee.

After being reported, a bill is placed on the calendar for floor consideration. A bill that has been reported by a committee generally cannot be considered on the floor until the committee report has been available to the members for three calendar days.

Floor Consideration of Measures

Calendars

Both the House and Senate have calendar systems by which the order of business on the floor is determined. There are two major calendars in the House: the Union calendar and the House calendar. The Union calendar governs the vast majority of public bills including revenue and appropriation measures. In the Senate, there is only one calendar: the Calendar of Business.

Consent Measures

In both chambers, measures may be considered out of calendar order by consent; normally this is done only with noncontroversial measures that are placed on the Consent calendar, considered on certain days, and passed by unanimous consent without debate. In the Senate on any day but Monday, any Senator may move to take a bill out of its regular order on the calendar.

House Consideration

In the House, it is possible to use one of two means to have a measure taken out of order to the floor. First, a special resolution or "rule" may be obtained from the Committee on Rules providing for expedited consideration of a measure. Such a rule limits debate on the measure to a specified amount of time and defines permissible amendments, if any. House rules require that all amendments be germane and that they be the same subject matter as the bill they propose to alter. If a member has been unsuccessful in convincing the committee reporting the bill to accept an amendment, or if he disagrees with the bill as reported, this is his opportunity to obtain floor consideration of an amendment. A modified open rule, which limits amendments by specifying which sections can be amended, will block floor consideration of an amendment unless specifically provided for in the rule. A closed rule prohibits any amendments on the floor. Rules are reported from the Rules Committee as House Resolutions and must be adopted by a majority vote of the House.

Second, a measure also may be considered out of calendar order through a motion and vote to suspend the rules. Such a motion may only be made on certain days and requires an affirmative vote of two-thirds of the members present.

The House has a parliamentary device thath enables it to act with a quorum of 100 instead of the usual 218; it is known as the Committee of the Whole House on the State of the Union. All measures on the Union calendar must be considered by the Committee of the Whole, usually five minutes each for the proponents and the opponents of the legislation. The Committee of the Whole then votes on the measure and reports it to the full House.

Once a measure is before the full House, it may be subject to further debate on the floor. Voting in the House may be in any of five ways: 1) "voice vote" where the chair determines the results of a vote on the volume of ayes and nays; 2) "division vote" where the members in favor and in opposition stand separately and are counted; 3) "teller vote" where the chair appoints tellers who count the votes for and against a bill; 4) "recorded vote" where the vote is taken by electronic device; and 5) "yea and nay vote" that requires each member to respond to the calling of the roll. A member also may vote "present."

After passage by the House, the "engrossed" bill is compiled, including any amendments made on the floor. At this time, the measure ceases to be a bill and becomes an "Act", although it often is referred to informally as a bill."

Senate Consideration

Senate floor consideration of measures has fewer procedural complexities than the House. A bill may be called up in its regular order on the calendar, or a separate motion may be made to consider the bill out of order. There is no rule for limiting debate unless a unanimous consent agreement is made. Upon obtaining the floor, senators may speak as long as they wish but not more than twice on any question in debate on the same day, without leave of the Senate. This rule gives rise to the practice of "filibustering," where those in opposition to the measure hold the floor continuously to prevent passage. Cloture, the closing of debate, can be obtained only by sixteen senators agreeing to the making of such a motion and a two-thirds vote of those present. All Senate measures are subject to unlimited debate and there is no requirement that amendments be germane (ie, be the same subject as the rest of the bill). A simple majority is needed for passage of a measure, and a vote may be taken by voice or roll call vote if so demanded by one-fifth of the senators present.

Resolution of Differing Versions

Because both the House and Senate must pass identical measures before legislation may go to the President, any differences between the House and Senate versions of the passed bills must be resolved. This may be accomplished in one of several ways. If the amendments are noncontroversial, the chamber to which the bill has been referred can simply accept the other chamber's amendments by unanimous consent. If the measures differ only in minor respects, the committees that had jurisdiction over the bills may informally work out an acceptable compromise. The chamber that first passed the bill then re-passes it with the mutually agreed upon amendments, and the second chamber then accepts them by unanimous consent.

If the amendments by the second chamber are extensive or controversial, a conference will be requested when the bill is returned to the first chamber. Each chamber appoints conferees who meet to eliminate differences between the bills. Such a conference committee cannot change portions of the bill that are not in dispute or cannot add additional provisions. If no agreement can be reached, the bill will die in conference. If agreement is reached, the conference committee issues a report of the decisions made and the reasons for them. The conference report must then be adopted by both chambers. Conference reports are privileged and are not subject to amendments on the floor. Once both chambers have passed identical versions of the measure, the bill is enrolled for presentation to the President.

Presidential Action

Once the enrolled bill is delivered to the White House, the President has ten days in which to act. If the President approves of the bill, he may sign it within that period. If he does not return the bill to the Congress within ten days (Sundays excepted), it will become law automatically without his signature. The President, however, may "pocket veto" a bill —if Congress adjourns during the ten day period so that the President cannot return the bill, and he does not sign it, it will not become law.

If the President vetoes a measure, it is returned to the chamber in which it originated along with a statement of his objections. A motion to consider a veto is privileged and is in order at any time. A two-thirds vote of the members present and voting is necessary to override a veto. If the first chamber does not vote to override, the measure dies. If the chamber does override, the other chamber also must approve the override by a two-thirds majority to have the bill become law.

Knowledge will forever govern ignorance, and a people that mean to be their own governors must arm themselves with the Power that knowledge brings.- James Madison

There was a time, not too long ago, when a legislative effort could successfully be predicated on anecdotal evidence. It was very common for witnesses testifying on health issues to support their positions by giving examples of how individual patients would be affected by the proposal at issue. Testimony, for example, would be heard that a named patient was deprived of needed care by the operation of a given Medicare provision. By using such real life examples to play to the sympathies of members of Congress, support for legislative provisions was garnered. Because of Congress' proclivity to act on the basis of such evidence, few organizations were willing to expend the resources necessary to develop detailed empirical data to support their proposals.

The press of the federal budget deficit has dramatically changed the nature of the information that Congress will enact legislation. While members of Congress still harbor sympathy for the tribulations of individual patients, such examples will generally not be sufficient to persuade them to act on a legislative matter. Instead, congressional committees now demand hard empirical evidence of the need for each new health care proposal. Furthermore, the cost of every proposed health amendment now is calculated by the Congressional Budget Office. These cost estimates then are weighed against the benefits of the amendment and against the cost and benefits of every other provision contained in the legislative package. Only those amendments that are justified on both policy and cost grounds are likely to find their way into law.

This new approach to legislative decision-making places a high premium on the development of empirical data to establish the rationale for an amendment. If physical therapists, for example, sought to increase the limitation on outpatient physical therapy services from $500 to $1,000 annually, they would have to carry the burden of demonstrating that the additional federal expenditure required by the increase would be offset by savings resulting from the amendment (eg, that the increased access to physical therapy the amendment would engender would reduce patients' needs for other, higher cost services paid for by Medicare; that the increase in the limitation is more important than other services currently funded by Medicare and that those other expenditures therefore should be reduced commensurately; or that the increase is important enough to justify the development of other sources of revenue). In any of these cases, the burden of proof would be on the physical therapists, and no legislation would be likely unless that burden could be sustained.

To put it simply, legislative initiatives advanced by physical therapists in the coming years will necessitate the expenditure of manpower and financial resources to secure the data required to establish the empirical cases for those initiatives. It will be important, therefore, for individual physical therapists to monitor closely their own practices so that when they are approached by the APTA to supply information to support a legislative endeavor they will be in a position to make the information available.

Congress' current reliance on empirical data does not mean that anecdotal evidence no longer has any use. Although such information may not sway a congressional committee, it may be effective particularly in persuading a member of Congress who represents the physical therapist or his patient that a particular amendment is worthwhile. Physical therapists should be prepared to convey examples based their own personal experiences to their representatives in the House and the Senate. In this fashion, the anecdotal evidence supplied by physical therapists complements and strengthens the policy and empirical cases presented by the APTA in Washington, DC.

Grassroots . . . the ultimate source of power. —William Safire

The most successful legislative campaigns are often those supported by vigorous grassroots lobbying. An effective grassroots effort entails voting constituents communicating their views on legislative proposals to their congressmen and senators. This form of lobbying is especially potent because the persons expressing their views are responsible for electing the legislators to Congress. As a result, those constituents who are willing to take the time to approach their congressmen on legislative matters generally will find that they have their rapt attention.

Communicating with a congressman or senator is an art form and there are several time-tested guidelines that will significantly enhance the effectiveness of a communication whether it be written or oral.

First, the presentation must be planned carefully and researched thoroughly. Constituents will generally find that they have but one meaningful opportunity to discuss an issue with a member of Congress so they must be prepared to make the best of it. A presentation that is inaccurate, rambling, or overly emotional may well be more harmful to the legislative effort than no communication at all. Furthermore, a poor presentation may discourage a legislator from entertaining a constituent's views on other matters in the future.

Proper preparation requires constituents to decide which issues to raise with their congressmen. Only the one or two highest priority matters should be raised at any given time. Weaving less important issues into the presentation may obfuscate the critical issues and give the legislator an opportunity to help on the lesser priority items and thereby avoid assisting on the often more difficult high priority items.

Once the issues have been identified, the constituent must become thoroughly versed in the issue as well as the proposed legislative solution. Complete familiarity with the policy arguments and data supporting the legislative endeavor also is essential. It is axiomatic that the arguments and data proffered at the grassroots level must not conflict with the positions being espoused by the profession's representatives.

An equally important facet of the preparatory process is a study of each of the members of Congress to whom a presentation will be made. Physical therapists, for example, will want to know whether the member sits on one of the committees that has jurisdiction over health legislation, whether the member has an active interest in health care in general and physical therapy in particular, and whether there is anything in the legislator's background that could make the presentation easier (eg, a member of his or her family was treated successfully by a physical therapist). Such information can be obtained from local media coverage of the politician, the member's office, acquaintances of the legislator, and from the APTA.

Second, whether the presentation is oral or written, it must define succinctly the problem and explain how physical therapists or patients are affected by that problem, state the proposed solution and explain how it rectifies the problem, and describe precisely what it is that the member of Congress should do (eg, vote for or against proposed legislation). Under all circumstances, keep it simple and direct.

Third, unless physical therapists know otherwise, they should assume that legislators know very little about physical therapy or the manner in which physical therapy services are furnished. Members of Congress have extremely large and diverse areas of responsibility and it is unrealistic to believe that they could be sufficiently familiar with physical therapy to be able to understand readily even those issues that appear to be simplistic to the physical therapist. The presentation should proceed logically and in laymen's terms; technical terms and professional jargon should be avoided.

Fourth, each presentation should identify the constituent and the nature of his or her interests. For example, if a physical therapist furnishes services in a rehabilitation agency, the presentation should include a concise explanation of how an agency operates, the kinds of patients seen, and the types of services provided. In addition, if appropriate, the physical therapist's association with APTA should be detailed, and the legislator should be requested to support the Association's proposals when they are advanced to him or her.

Fifth, the action that legislators are asked to take must be reasonable. In fashioning the relief they seek, physical therapists should be sensitive to the diverse political, economic, and demographic interests each legislator must try to accommodate in the enactment of legislation. Pains should be taken to explain why a vote for the proposed legislation is a good political vote for the legislator (eg, the bill helps the elderly and the Congressman represents a district with a high aged census).

Sixth, it is important to appreciate the great time constraints under which members of Congress and their staffs must labor. The typical legislator has full committee and subcommittee assignments, caucus and party responsibilities, district obligations, and an onerous schedule of meetings with other members, lobbyists, and constituents. As someone seeking to pique a legislator's interest in yet another issue, the physical therapist's presentation should take these time pressures into account. The member's time should not be wasted on frivolous matters or matters not requiring legislative intervention. Where possible, contacts with members should be made in the congressional district where they generally have more time. The constituent's professional association should ensure that the proper contacts are made on Capitol Hill. If physical therapists have stated their positions orally, the legislator should be provided with written material to which they can refer at a later time.

Seventh, a Member of Congress or staff person should never be threatened with reprisals, political or otherwise, if the support sought is not forthcoming. Threats do not work, and they can be highly detrimental. At best, the legislator will not be receptive to future proposals advanced by the maker of the threat. At worst, the member may work actively to defeat the legislation the threatener wants.

Eighth, contacts on legislative matters must be made in a timely fashion (eg, when hearings begin in a committee or before a bill is scheduled for a vote in committee or on the floor).

Ninth, appreciation should always be expressed for the member's efforts even if they ultimately are not successful.

> *Politics should be the part-time profession of every citizen.*
> —Dwight D. Eisenhower

Many people are loath to become involved in politics but they should not be. Our representative form of government is predicated on the power of the electorate to vote into office those congressmen and senators who best represent the views of the voters and who are best able to protect their interests. It is a constitutional right, not a burden to be avoided, to work to elect representatives in Congress.

Working on an member's election or re-election campaign is an excellent way to establish a useful personal relationship with the legislator. Constituents can be helpful to members in a number of ways including organizing receptions and fundraisers, canvassing voters, making telephone calls on behalf of the campaign committee, and working at the polls. Physical therapists may make their expertise available to the legislator. They can organize tours of the health care facilities in which they provide services and furnish the candidate with opportunities to meet employees and patients. In addition, physical therapists can advise candidates on campaign strategies and policy issues concerning elderly or disabled persons. Activities such as these can prove to be invaluable when the time comes to talk to a member about an important legislative issue. The most successful relationships are forged when a constituent "does not need something" from the legislator. Any legislator will be more receptive to requests from individuals who volunteer to help at a time when the individual is not looking for a favor than they will be to requests from persons who offer their aid only when the person needs help from the member.

In deciding who to support and assist, it is important to check each candidate's voting records on issues of interest to the constituent. Physical therapists, for example, would be interested in votes on Medicare and Medicaid issues, particularly those legislative proposals in which physical therapists and the APTA have expressed a position.

Individuals must also be careful not to follow traditional party lines blindly. The decision as to which candidate to support should be made on the basis of views on issues of importance to physical therapists and not on the party label the candidate wears. It makes little sense, for example, to work to re-elect a member of Congress who has not supported physical therapists on legislative issues simply because that candidate is a Republican.

Physical therapists also may participate in the political process by making financial contributions to the candidates of their choice. This may be accomplished either through personal contributions made directly to the candidate or through contributions to action committees such as those sponsored by the APTA ("APT-CAC"— or the National Association of Rehabilitation Agencies ("NARA-PAC"). For several reasons, contributions made through such committees often will prove to be more effective than individual private contributions. First, contributions made to such PACs are combined with those of other physical therapists and presented to members of Congress as an expression of support from the sponsoring organization and its members. A PAC's ability to join several separate contributions to make a large contribution makes it a more potent force than the one from an individual who cannot afford to make such a large contribution. Second, legislators will see contributions from the PAC as an indication that they enjoy the broad support of the physical therapy profession and not just a single physical therapist. As a result, they may be more disposed to help when the need arises. And finally, as explained by Senator David Durenberger before the Senate Rules Committee on January 26, 1983:

> Political action committees have had a positive impact on the political process in their own way. Through their own organizing efforts, tens of thousands of American citizens have become active, contributing stakeholders in the political process for the first time in their lives. These contributions open the door to individual contributions of time and financial resources in the future. Candidates seeking PAC funds

have been forced to go outside the traditional Washington "money community" and explain their views to a broader cross section of their constituents.

Getting involved in politics either through campaign work or a financial contribution is not untoward conduct; it is a way of ensuring that this country's representative form of government works as it was intended by the framers of the Constitution.

> *It is not knowledge of ways and means we lack, it is the will to put them into effect.*
>
> —Alfred Vanderbilt

The ultimate success of physical therapists in securing important legislative objectives depends in large part on the willingness of individual physical therapists to participate in the legislative and political processes at the grassroots level. Physical therapists should not be reticent to utilize their experiences and expertise to this end. To paraphrase Spinoza, the legislature abhors a vacuum, and if physical therapists do not move to fill that void they can be certain that their adversaries will.

CHAPTER 9

Alternative Delivery Systems for Physical Therapists

Michael Weinper, MPH, PT

It wasn't that long ago, so it seems, that physical therapy services were delivered without much concern over the source of payment. After all, physical therapy was a valuable and necessary component of any health care delivery system; thus the care warranted payment. Various payment sources, including Medicare, Medicaid, workers' compensation, and indemnity insurance, covered these services. Health maintenance organizations (HMOs) also provided physical therapy services in their encapsulated delivery models.

Then, in the late 1960s, strange things began to happen. The Medicare administration observed what appeared to be gross improprieties in services rendered to recipients of that program. Health care costs began to spiral upward at a much greater rate than other components of the cost of living index. And with the new-found profits in health care came a proliferation of physicians and hospitals. With this proliferation health care competition was born.

When examining the impact of alternative health care delivery systems on the delivery of physical therapy services, one must understand the operating characteristics and historical background of each of the models.

Indemnity Plans

The first health insurance plans in this country were of the indemnity, or fee for service type. Organized labor played an important role in the provision of health care benefits to employees of organizations with collective bargaining units. Insurance was purchased to provide health benefits on an

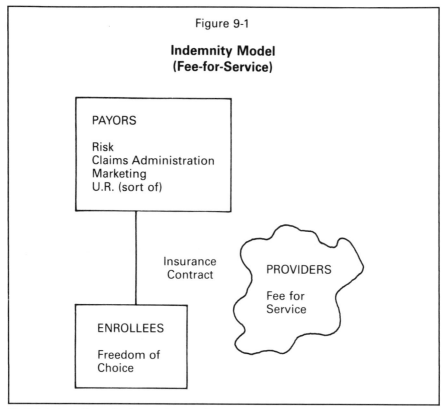

Figure 9-1

**Indemnity Model
(Fee-for-Service)**

PAYORS

Risk
Claims Administration
Marketing
U.R. (sort of)

Insurance
Contract

PROVIDERS

Fee for
Service

ENROLLEES

Freedom of
Choice

Fig 9-1. Indemnity, or fee-for-service, mode.

"as needed" basis by the insured. To limit risk of the insurance company, *deductibles* and *copayment* concepts were developed. Deductibles are the "first dollar" expenses that are the responsibility of the insured rather than the insuror. Copayments or coinsurance are the portion of covered benefits paid by the insured after the deductible is met. Both serve as a disincentive for the insured to obtain services. An example is the traditional 80%/20% benefit where the insuror pays 80% and the insured pays a copayment of 20%.

Although this traditional form of insurance provided the patient with free choice of providers (eg, physician, hospital, therapist), it did not and does not contain many components to prevent overutilization of services. In recent years, many indemnity plans have instituted second opinions before delivery of high-cost elective services. To keep premiums at a competitive level with other insurance types, larger deductible amounts have been instituted, thereby limiting risk by the insuror to later expenses. Higher deductibles and copayments provide a disincentive for routine or nonemergency services, because the patient is responsible for greater out-of-pocket expenses.

In summary, indemnity, or fee-for-service, insurance provides the patient a free choice of provider with few constraints on the delivery of services. This model is illustrated in Figure 9-1.

Health Maintenance Organizations

Contrary to the perceptions of many, the concept of HMOs, or prepaid programs, is not a new or recent development. The earliest prepaid plans can be traced to the 1920s when Dr. Donald Ross established a health care program in a railroad settlement in Canada. He saw the need for the delivery of services in the railroad and lumber industries where settlements were remote from medical care facilities. He was joined in 1929 by another physician, Dr. Clifford Loos, and the Ross-Loos Medical Group was formed in California. These individuals received much criticism and censure from their local medical associations for this break from the traditional fee-for-service delivery model in which the employer prepaid for any and all services that might be required by its employees.

The nation's largest non-profit HMO, Kaiser Permanente, was founded in 1938 to benefit the Kaiser employees constructing the Grand Coulee Dam in Washington state. This program achieved great success and was expanded to other areas where Kaiser had employees. The program was limited to their employees until 1946 when it was first offered to the public. Now known as the Kaiser Foundation Health Plan, this HMO provides services to over 4,762,000 members in ten states and the District of Columbia.

While Kaiser grew steadily throughout the years, the HMO concept did not gain popularity throughout the country until the 1970s. In fact, in the late 1960s while the HMO concept had been in existence for nearly fifty years there were only 35 prepaid plans nationwide. This number grew to 230 in 1980 and 480 in 1985 (Tab. 9-1 and Fig. 9-2). Most significant is the birth of 143 plans (42.4% increase) between 1984 and 1985.

This dramatic change was brought on by many factors including the rapid escalation of health care costs, a glut of physicians and hospitals, and an increasing cost to employers who pay for the majority of health benefits in this country. The HMO concept, through its "pay one price" image, became popular with those government, labor, business and health care professions who had varying needs for this form of health care delivery. Employers were concerned over escalating costs of providing benefits. Labor unions, wishing to represent the needs of their members, also realized management's limitations on providing a fixed level of benefits in light of escalating costs. Labor's concern was simple. If employers couldn't afford to keep up with the cost of coverage, benefits to the employee would be reduced, weakening labor's benefit to their members. Both federal and state governments, which represent major purchasers of health benefits for their employees, also were concerned with the expense of providing benefits to their employees. With the proliferation of physicians in this country, solo and small group practices often were declining in profitability; therefore, the HMO provided a safe haven for guaranteed employment with reasonable compensation and limited working hours.

In 1973, the HMO Assistance Act provided federal grants for the development and expansion of this delivery model. The 1310 Mandate developed a federal qualification that allowed HMOs to require employers to offer a

TABLE 9-1. SUMMARY OF HMO GROWTH 1981-1988

	JUNE 1981	JUNE 1982	JUNE 1983	JUNE 1984	JUNE 1985	JUNE 1986	JUNE 1987	JUNE 1988
NUMBER OF PLANS:								
TOTAL NUMBER OF PLANS	243	265	280	306	393	595	662	643
PERCENT CHANGE FROM PREVIOUS YEAR	3%	9.1%	5.7%	9.3%	28.9%	51.3%	11.2%	−2.8%
NUMBER OF NEW PLANS	20	38	24	40	92	217	95	32
PERCENT OF PLANS	8.2%	14.3%	8.6%	13.1%	23.4%	217%*	14.3%	4.9%
ENROLLMENT:								
TOTAL ENROLLMENT	10,266,172	10,831,229	12,490,780	15,140,756	18,893,607	23,663,626	28,587,119	31,366,031
PERCENT CHANGE FROM PREVIOUS YEAR	12.8%	5.5%	15.3%	21.2%	24.8%	25.2%	20.8%	9.7%
PLAN SIZE:								
AVERAGE SIZE	42,238	40,873	44,610	49,479	48,075	39,771	48,183	48,781
PERCENT CHANGE FROM PREVIOUS YEAR	9.6%	−3.3%	9.1%	10.9%	−2.8%	−17.2%	21.1%	1.2%
PERCENT OF MEMBERS IN PLANS WITH 100,000 OR MORE MEMBERS	61%	61%	60%	58%	56%	52%	53%	56%

REPRINTED WITH PERMISSION OF INTERSTUDY, EXCELSIOR, MN
NATIONAL HMO CENSUS

*increase from 6/85-6/86

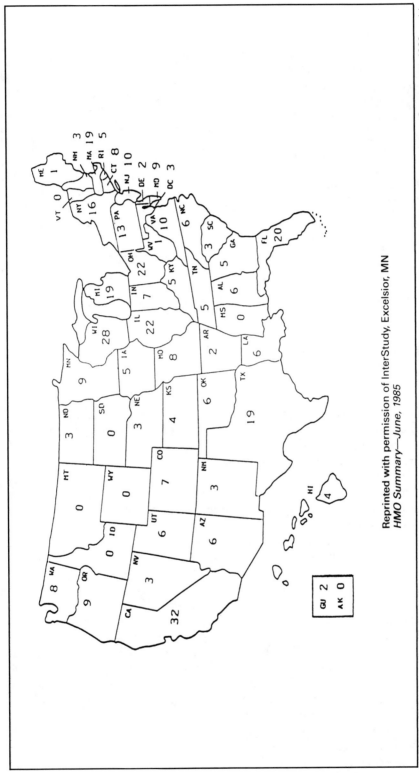

Reprinted with permission of InterStudy, Excelsior, MN
HMO Summary—June, 1985

Fig 9-2. Numbers of health maintenance organizations by state, June 1985. (Reprinted from *Health Maintenance Organization Summary—1988,* with permission of Interstudy, Excelsion, MN.

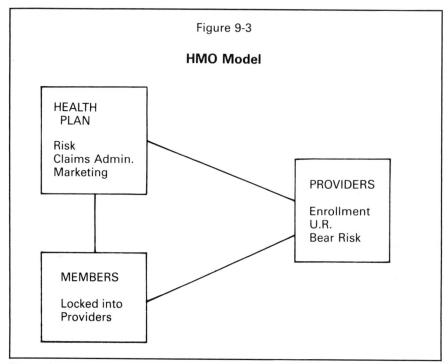

Fig 9-3. Health maintenance organization model.

prepaid plan if the employer had health care as a benefit and more than 25 employees. This mandate created an increased marketplace in which the HMO model prospered.

HMOs have become an effective delivery model because they help contain costs by having providers of care share in some aspect of risk. (Fig. 9-3) The objective is to minimize the unnecessary utilization of medical care, controlling the overall cost. Capitation can simply be defined as a fixed payment to a provider per enrollee. This payment is made regardless of whether or not that enrollee receives any services.

An HMO differs from the traditional indemnity model in several ways. A Health Maintenance Organization is actually responsible for the provision of care and it must assure accessibility to care. Members or enrollees are limited to receiving services from a specific pool of providers and thus have been restricted from a freedom of choice of providers as seen in the traditional mode. Payment to the providers is often on a capitation or prospective basis, thereby giving control of the health care dollar expenditure to the physician who can benefit from proper utilization of services. An HMO provides services for a fixed monthly payment that is prepaid and which does not vary according to the amount of services obtained by each member. An HMO must provide a comprehensive health program for both hospital and physician services. Members are "locked in" to the plan for a specific time. The capitation concept shifts the risk from the payor to the provider who then becomes financially responsible for the patient's care.

HMOs can be of two primary types. Federally qualified HMOs must provide a standard menu of full benefits to its members. Non-federally qualified HMOs can tailor their benefit packages to meet the needs of their purchasers. Federally qualified plans also differ from non-federally qualified plans inasmuch as they may not use experience in setting rates. That is to say that federally qualified plans cannot give better rates to groups who have a history of "healthy" members. Non-federally qualified plans can accordingly provide an "experience" rating which can take utilization and morbidity experiences into account in modifying premiums for certain classifications of members.

HMOs can also be classified into four different models. Models describe the predominant structure or practice style of the plan. The "staff model" is an HMO that delivers health services through a physician group that is controlled by the HMO plan. The "group model" is an HMO that contracts with one independent group practice to provide health services to its members. The "independent practice association model (IPA)" is a plan with one or more of the following characteristics:

1. The HMO contracts directly with the physicians in independent practice;
2. The HMO contracts with one or more associations of physicians in independent practice;
3. The HMO contracts with one or more multispecialty group practices but the plan is organized predominantly around solo/single-specialty practices.

Last, the "network model" is an HMO that contracts with two or more independent group practices, possibly including a staff group, to provide health services. Although the network may contain a few solo practices, it is organized predominantly around groups.

Each of these models may utilize physical therapy in different ways. The staff model traditionally is large enough to support the employment of physical therapists to deliver rehabilitative care. This same model is noted often in the group practice. Dependent on the size and needs of group practices, the network model may utilize a physical therapist on a capitation or a fee-for-service basis or, in fact, may provide it through physical therapists employed by one or more of the independent group practices. The IPA model typically provides physical therapy through independent physical therapists on either a capitation or a fee-for-service basis but also may utilize physical therapists employed by physicians within specialty practices that are part of the IPA.

Just as the HMO concept discourages utilization through its prepaid form of compensation, the IPA delivery model tends to provide physical therapy services at lower utilization rates than seen in the indemnity or Preferred Provider Organization (PPO) models. Generally, an emphasis is placed on wellness, and physical therapists are involved often in preventive aspects of care including the use of proper body mechanics, self-care techniques, prenatal and postnatal exercise instruction and other health education functions intended to decrease the need for acute or subacute care. When an injury or illness requires specific physical therapy services, the HMO model has been observed to provide less direct care and a greater emphasis on patients caring for themselves, whenever possible. This phenomenon has not been documented through utilization review data, as no such information existed in the literature for the utilization of physical therapy services by diagnostic category in various health care delivery models. This phenomenon, however, has been described by many therapists working within the HMO models or contracting with such programs. Another factor lending itself to decreased physical therapy utilization is the financial disincentive for physicians who have been capitated for all services to have to "spend" funds for physical therapy services when it may be perceived that such services are elective and may be unnecessary. Accordingly, physical therapists often find themselves in the role of an educator rather than a clinician delivering hands-on care.

Physical therapists who contract on a fee-for-service basis with HMOs frequently describe a decline, both in the frequency of referrals of patients and the frequency and duration of authorized treatments for diagnoses as compared with their traditional indemnity experience. These comments are not intended as a criticism of the HMO model, but rather as an observation. In the absence of objective outcome information by diagnosis in the comparative models, any critique would be arbitrary at best.

An informal survey of physical therapists in states that have experienced a proliferation of HMO enrollment in recent years has revealed a decline in their practices' pool of indemnity-insured patients. As these therapists have investigated the decline of referrals from their referring sources, they have learned that the referring practitioners have also experienced similar declines in their practices. Accordingly, physical therapists must consider participation in HMO on either an employment basis or, if they wish to remain independent, on a fee-for-service or capitation basis.

If physical therapists wish to participate in a capitated program, they need to be aware of several factors that can affect the financial reasonableness of such a relationship. The first question is who controls the referral and utilization of physical therapy services. This question cannot be answered without also considering who is financially at risk for the expense. If physicians control the referral and utilization but physical therapists are locked into providing services for a fixed capitation amount (at risk), physical therapists may find that they are providing great quantities of service at a low rate per visit. Yet, if the referring providers are at financial risk, physical therapists can expect a lower rate of utilization of physical therapy services than would otherwise be anticipated.

Another concern for physical therapists participating in capitated programs is the concept of stop-loss. Stop-loss is best equated to a form of insurance where providers (in this case physical therapists) are assured of a limited amount of services that will be provided for the capitated fee. This provision does not come free of charge to providers and, in fact, often is "purchased" by physical therapists through a decreased capitation amount than would otherwise be provided. Stop-loss features can be applied on an individual case basis or an aggregate basis for the overall utilization of physical therapy services by the group. Stop-loss provisions can be very beneficial in limiting a physical therapist's risk to providing a high number of services in return for a low level of capitated compensation.

Preferred Provider Organization

Compared with the history of indemnity programs and HMOs, the Preferred Provider Organization (PPO) concept is rather new. Unfortunately, the acronym for this model has taken on many meanings depending on who is doing the describing, whether it be insurance companies, providers, or patients. In fact, because the arrangements for PPOs are so diverse, it has it's been said "when you've seen one PPO...you've seen one PPO." Nevertheless, a PPO can be described as follows:

An organization of fee-for-service providers who have a contractual arrangement to provide health care services at a negotiated rate to a defined pool of patients who have freedom of choice of provider but have economic incentive to utilize PPO member providers.

At first glance, this definition can be overwhelming; yet when broken into its components, the definition should become clear.

Organization of Providers. The delivery system can either be formed by providers, organized by a third party such as an insurance company, or developed by a self-insured employer. There are contractual and operational links between the providers and the organizing entity.

Fee-for-Service. The provider's remuneration is based on the units of service provided. The price of each unit of service generally is determined through negotiations between the provider and the payer. Unit prices may differ for the various purchasers of the PPO services.

Contracts. Contracts are negotiated and executed to determine the specific terms of the relationships between the parties.(Fig.9-4) Contracts can exist between the PPO organizing entity and each of its providers, the PPO and the payer, or the payer and each provider.

The contracts normally will contain provisions dealing with:
- the range of services to be provided
- compensation arrangements and prices
- utilization review policies and procedures
- inspection of records
- insurance and general liability issues
- dispute resolution processes
- referrals to non-PPO providers
- termination, contract renewal, and price negotiations

Negotiated Rates. Most purchasers of care will not be satisfied with the providers' routine pricing structure; however, it should not be assumed that the negotiated price always reflects a discount. Other benefits to the payor such as a utilization review program may satisfy the payor that cost savings will be in the scope and duration of services provided, rather than in a cost savings on a per unit of service basis. A statewide PPO for physical therapy in California, the Physical Therapy Provider Network, Inc (PTPN), has, in several cases, negotiated rates with payers that provide compensation to the

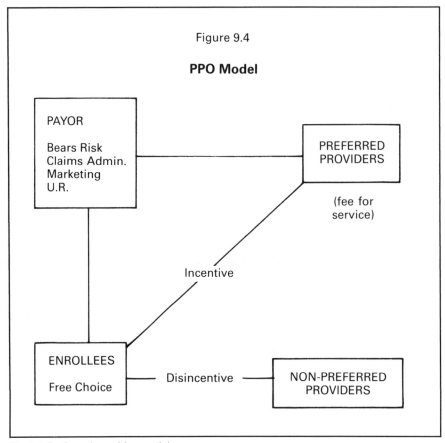

Fig 9-4. Preferred provider model.

participating physical therapist at no discount from their normal rate structure.

Defined Pool of Patients. This defined pool consists of the subscribers, employees, or insureds who have enrolled in a special benefit program that directs them to the PPO providers.

Free Choice. In contrast to HMO patients, PPO patients may use the services of any provider within the PPO network and receive full benefits. The patient also may use the services of a non-PPO provider; however, a significant additional payment by the patient will normally be required.

Economic Incentive. Although the patient can use the services of non-PPO providers, it will be costly to do so. Increased deductibles and copayments are the usual penalties. The payer must agree to and the provider should insist on a well-designed set of penalties or financial incentives to keep the patient within the PPO network. The absence of financial incentives for the patient to "stay within the network" dilutes the advantages for physical therapists participating in these programs.

When examining the PPO concept from a historical prespective, its roots can be traced to California. (Fig.9-5) In 1982, the California legislature

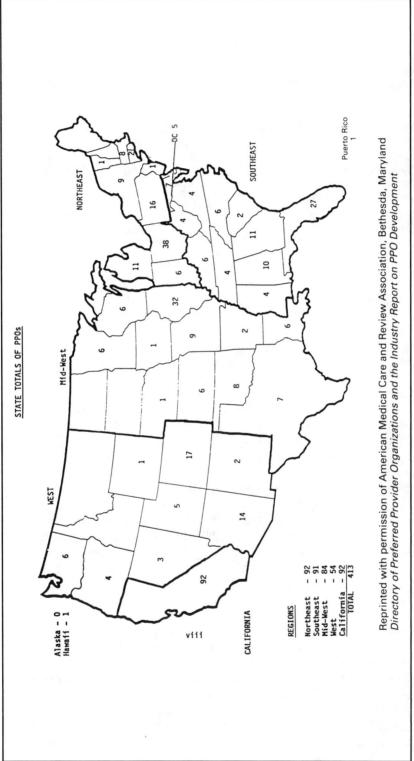

Fig 9-5. Development of preferred provider organizations from 1980 and before to June 1, 1988. (Reprinted from *Directory of Preferred Provider Organizations and the Industry Report on PPO Development*, with permission of American Medical Care Review Association, Bethesda, MD.

Reprinted with permission of American Medical Care and Review Association, Bethesda, Maryland *Directory of Preferred Provider Organizations and the Industry Report on PPO Development*

STATE TOTALS OF PPOs

REGIONS

Northeast	– 92
Southeast	– 91
Mid-West	– 84
West	– 54
California	– 92
TOTAL	413

Alaska – 0
Hawaii – 1

Puerto Rico 1

NORTHEAST

SOUTHEAST

Mid-West

WEST

CALIFORNIA

DC 5

viii

TABLE 9-2
Summary of Sponsorship

Category	Number June, 1988	June, 1987
Other Insurance Carrier	153	121
Physician-Hospital	119	113
Physicians	86	105
Blue Cross/Blue Shield Combined	61	59
Hospitals	63	64
Investor	50	47
Third Party Administrator	29	25
HMOs	18	18
Self Insured Employer	10	9
Others	71	9
Total	660	570

passed Assembly Bill 799 that allowed MediCal (Medicaid in California) to contract statewide with a selective number of hospitals. Subsequent legislation, Assembly Bill 3480, permitted the development of a new health care delivery system known as the PPO. With these statutes, the state of California chose selective contracting as the preferred approach to health care cost containment. This concept allows insurance companies and other payers to contract selectively with providers of care (physicians, hospitals, physical therapists, and other health professionals or providers). Subsequently, Blue Cross of California commenced contractual negotiations to create a network of providers for its Prudent Buyer Plan in March of 1983. As a result of this legislation, a wide spectrum of payers and providers began to establish contracting entities to participate in this new, alternative health care delivery system marketplace. According to statistics published by the American Medical Care and Review Association (AMCRA), of the 660 PPOs reporting throughout the country in 1988, 639 were of operational status and 21 claimed to be preoperational. (Fig.9-6) A summary of sponsorship of these organizations can be found in Table 2. The AMCRA reports a total membership of 33,936,000 for PPOs reporting data in June 1988. Some predictions anticipate growth of enrollment to between 40 to 60 million enrollees by 1990.

The PPO concept, as of this writing, is too new to comment on regarding physical therapy utilization patterns. The PPO model encourages referral to providers within the system while also providing financial disincentives to patients who seek services outside the preferred network. Patients maintain the freedom to obtain their physical therapy services in any location; however, some learn soon the financial advantages of higher reimbursement rates when obtaining services through a preferred physical therapist. Generally, all provider contracts contain a provision that states "referrals to other practitioners will be made only to other network providers." Although this clause should maintain the network's integrity, the burden still lies with patients to

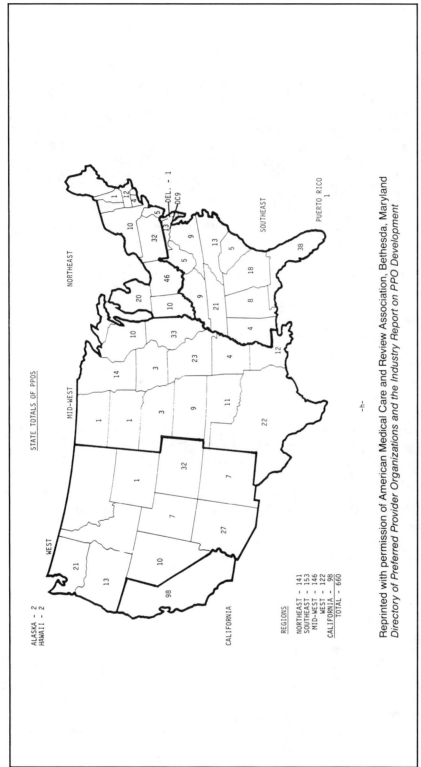

Fig 9-6. State totals of preferred provider organization. (Reprinted from *Directory of Preferred Provider Organizations and the Industry Report on PPO Development*, with permission of American Medical Care and Review Association, Bethesda, MD.

ensure that they stay within the network when there is a need for outpatient physical therapy services.

Unlike the HMO model where capitation may have a financial impact on the referring practitioner, the PPO referring practitioner is not financially affected by the frequency of referrals to physical therapy or other services. To prevent runaway expenses in PPO programs, utilization review programs have been developed to identify services provided by practitioners outside the scope of "community standards." The presence of a utilization review program in other settings has been found to create what has been known as the "sentinel effect." This phenomenon is seen often in situations where providers know that their performance is being monitored and thereby decrease their provision of services.

As physical therapy networks mature in their data collection processes, a significant new database will be developed that may provide the basis for determining prospective payment of outpatient physical therapy services.

Physical Therapy Provider Network: A Case Study

In 1985, the nation's first statewide PPO for physical therapists became operational. The Physical Therapy Provider Network, Inc. (PTPN), was developed to meet the needs of physical therapists in independent practice who wish to participate in this new health care marketplace.

PTPN is a professional corporation that is owned, in part, by each of the participating offices. The founders of PTPN determined that the needs of independent physical therapists were not being met in other models that had been developed. The objective of PTPN was and is to demonstrate to payers the financial and qualitative advantages of directing their patients to the independent physical therapists who participate in this unique network. The contracting focus of PTPN was aimed at the following five major market segments:

Insurors. Many insurance companies now are offering preferred product lines that can benefit from an outpatient physical therapy component.

Self-Insureds. Many self-insured employers, labor union trust funds, and third party administrators currently negotiate arrangements with providers of care.

Workers' Compensation. A potentially large market exists where the physical therapist can deliver quality services to workers' compensation payers. Physical therapy represents a major opportunity to control expenses through a comprehensive system for treating injured workers under a controlled utilization review system.

Health Maintenance Organizations. As discussed earlier, some HMOs utilize IPAs or networks for the provision of various health benefits including physical therapy.

PPO Networks. This market includes the PPOs formed by other providers (hospitals, physicians, physician-hospital combinations, and foundations for medical care). A physical therapy network can "piggyback" with these entities to form a comprehensive health benefit program.

PTPN has established membership criteria by which to determine eligibility of physical therapy offices interested in membership. These criteria include, the following:

1. Owned entirely by licensed physical therapists who render services free of the administrative control of the employer;
2. Maintains at its own expense an office and the necessary equipment to provide an adequate program of physical therapy services;
3. Employs only all physical therapists who are graduates of an entry-level program accredited by an agency recognized by the United States Department of Education, the Council on Postsecondary Accreditation or the equivalent;
4. Has a location certified by the Medicare program as independent physical therapy practice or "free-standing" rehabilitation agency;
5. Is owned by physical therapists who each have a minimum of three years' clinical experience;
6. Has physical therapy evaluations, treatment plans, and re-evaluations performed and documented by licensed physical therapists;
7. Has staffing ratios of aides or assistants that limit the overutilization of support personnel;
8. Does not restrict practices to a particular age, category, or specialty.

PTPN, in its design, also has developed limitations on the number of participating offices to avoid antitrust issues and provide financial benefits to its members through increased referrals.

Since its inception, PTPN has enrolled 145 offices throughout California and has contracted with insurance companies, self-insured employers, workers' compensation insurance companies, third party administrators, and health maintenance organizations representing over 1.5 million enrollees.

Exclusive Provider Organizations

In addition to creating the PPO concept in California, Assembly Bill 3480 developed an exclusive provider organization plan (EPO). The EPOs require beneficiaries to stay within the network to receive benefits; however, unlike the HMOs where the enrollee must choose a primary care physician, the patient has a freedom of choice of any provider within the network. This "lock in" provision establishes control for the provider because it restricts enrollees from seeking services outside the network. This model is of greater benefit to the providers within the network because utilization of the network's providers is guaranteed.

While not yet popular, this model will gain in acceptance as it offers the plan participant the freedom of choice within the network and it benefits the participating providers by limiting the choices of the enrollee to participating providers. The EPOs also may provide for an easier evaluation of process, outcome and cost because of the inability of the enrollee to receive services

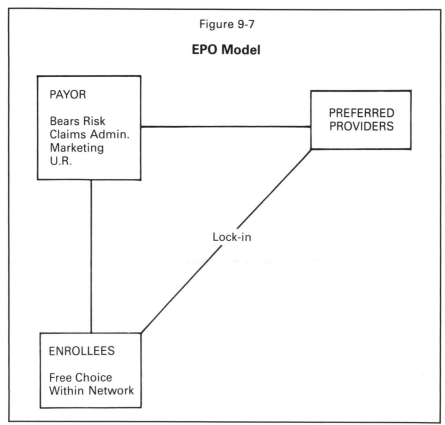

Fig 9-7. Exclusive provider organization model.

outside the network and the ease of obtaining data. This model is illustrated in Figure 9-7.

Discussion

The growth and acceptance of the HMOs, PPOs, and potentially EPOs, appear to reflect the concern purchasers have over the escalating costs of health care. These alternative models have demonstrated the ability to contain health care costs. More important, these models have been accepted by the recipients of care in each of the models.

On the contrary, many health care providers have voiced opposition to participating in the HMOs, PPOs, and EPOs. Providers are concerned about their future ability to profit in these systems and to make health care decisions independent of other influences, such as utilization review, second opinions, and nonpayment for non-covered services.

Payers have become involved in provider contracting as a means of staying competitive in this ever-changing marketplace. The HMOs and PPOs have changed the way that payors design, market, and administer their benefits programs. The HMOs are shifting the risk to the providers through capitation forms of payment. Physicians often are placed at risk for physical therapy services and then must decide whether it is "financially feasible" and necessary to provide physical therapy services or whether the patient's condition will improve without treatment.

The PPOs have grown in popularity as many large group health insurors have lost significant shares of business to the HMOs, Blue Cross-Blue Shield organizations, and employers who have elected to become self-insured for health benefits. The PPOs offer programs that can avoid the disadvantages of the HMOs through freedom of choice of provider; no financial disincentives for the referral of patients; and the perception, but not the reality, on which traditional health care continues to live. Unlike the HMOs that require patients to remain within the plan, the PPOs offer a dual option that allows patients either to remain in the plan or to obtain service outside the plan by paying a larger part of the expenses.

Critics of the PPO concept question the cost containment component in light of weak or nonexistent utilization review programs. The future success of the PPOs will be dependent not only on negotiated rates for service but on controls on the volume of services rendered by providers. As there is a segment of the population who does not wish to participate in prepaid plans, the PPOs and EPOs should experience a significant growth at the expense of indemnity programs.

Physical therapists must consider participation in these alternative health care delivery systems in order to survive. That is not to say that they should enter every program that seeks their participation. Physical therapists must be able to identify their costs of providing services and their desired profit margins. The following list of questions is presented as food for thought when contracting opportunities arise.

The physical therapist, prior to entering into a contractual relationship, should ask the following:

1. What are my goals for this practice?
2. What are my capacities/limitations to provide services?
3. Who is the payer?
4. Is the payer financially sound?
5. Who are the payers' clients (e.g., other insurance companies, employers)?
6. Who are the enrollees (demographic information)? How many enrollees are there in the program?
7. Is there a referral physician network? Must the physician refer to me?
8. How many other participating physical therapists are in the program?
9. Does the patient have a financial incentive to see me?
10. How do I find out if the patient is eligible for services?
11. Must prior authorization be given by the primary care physician, the referring physician (primary or specialist), the health plan?
12. Must I have a specific authorization document?
13. Must the authorization document be attached to my billing?
14. Is there a benefit limit on the number of physical therapy visits permitted?
15. Is there a benefit limit on the duration of services provided?

16. What are the copayments and deductibles?
17. What is the rate or basis of payment?
18. Will the payment be the lesser of the negotiated rate or my billed charges?
19. How soon must I submit my bills?
20. How soon will I be paid?
21. Does interest apply to late payments?
22. Who do I call about claims issues?
23. What are my rights if a claim is denied?
24. Can I collect from the patient if the payer does not pay?
25. Can I bill the patient for non-covered services?
26. At what rate can I bill the patient for non-covered services?
27. Can I bill and keep secondary insurance the patient may have?
28. How are contract disputes settled?
29. When does the contract terminate?
30. Can I terminate the contract early if I am dissatisfied?

The above list is not intended to be all inclusive but rather to offer the physical therapist a set of issues to consider prior to signing on the dotted line.

As many of these questions are quite technical, physical therapists may wish to join with other physical therapists in a PPO structure that meets their needs. The PPOs have demonstrated their ability to aid the provider in answering many of these questions, and in obtaining higher rates of compensation compared with the rates negotiated by individual therapists. It has often been said that there is strength in numbers, and physical therapists will benefit best by participating in alternative health care delivery systems if they follow the lead that has been established by physicians and hospital groups.

In conclusion, the participation by physical therapists in health care delivery systems no longer is a simple proposition. For physical therapists to prosper in this emerging marketplace, they must become more sophisticated and more knowledgeable about the costs of services, abilities, goals, and needs. Physical therapists who believe they can succeed just by being a good clinician will learn the painful truth that "it just ain't so....anymore".

CHAPTER 10

Information Management: The Technological Revolution

Jane Walter, EdD, PT

Four distinct innovations in information machines of the 1870s and 1880s —the Remington typewriter, the cash register, the William Burroughs printing adder and the Herman Hellerith punch-card tabulating equipment — laid the groundwork for information processing.[1] Each machine represented an advance in technology in which human error was reduced and information was stored efficiently. Today, when we talk about information technology we are talking about the use of computer technology to collect, sort and store information. Information management, however, requires more than a network of computer hardware. Information systems are found within organizations such as business, education, associations, and foundations. Information management requires a management system and human engineering to determine the manner in which information will be collected, stored, and retrieved. Furthermore, it requires a systematic planning process to assure that each component of an organization and each phase of the organization's development will fit into the system. Richard Nolan of Harvard Business School has defined six stages of growth of information management within an organization. These six stages are: initiation, contagion, control, integration, data administration, and maturity.[2] Every organization in which physical therapy education, research, or practice takes place no doubt is at a different stage of growth in information management. Organizations may have developed systems that intimately involved physical therapists in the planning of an information system serving the needs of the profession, or they may have developed a program that can be compatible with those needs. It is likely that an organization's first goal is to develop a system that supports the primary mission of the organization and the degree to which physical therapy is affected is the degree to which physical therapy education, research, or practice is a part of that mission. As a profession, physical therapy is in the beginning stages of growth (initiation, contagion) from an information management perspective, although in isolated cases information management has been integrated into specific education, research or practice arenas. As a profession, our challenge is to infuse enthusiasm for information technology by demonstrating its value in collecting, storing, sorting, handling, disseminating, and analyzing physical therapy information.

Within the context of information management, computer technology often has promoted the development of informational systems, and an understanding of the role of computers in a particular organization or profession often leads to an understanding of the degree of technological growth in that organization or profession. In this chapter I will explore the use of computers in physical therapy and the growth of information management within the profession and the professional association —the American Physical Therapy Association (APTA).

The introduction of the integrated circuit in 1959 led to the development of the computer chip that ended the first modern computer generation as "vacuum tubes, punched cards and machine codes [gave] way to second-generation transistors, magnetic tape and procedural languages in computer design and operation."[3] The development of the computer chip[1] and the computer language Beginner's All-Purpose Symbolic Instruction Code (BASIC) as a variation of FORTRAN in 1965 revolutionized the computer industry in that computers were now manageable in size, language, and cost. The first commercial minicomputer was produced in 1964 by Digital.[3] By 1967, the third generation of computers was "underway, with integrated circuits, floppy disks and nonprocedural languages becoming prominent in computer construction and usage."[3] The development of the Apple II personal computer (Apple) and the TRS-80 microcomputer (Radio Shack) in 1977 and the IBM personal computer in 1980 ushered in the personal computer[3] which now has become accessible to physical therapists in a variety of work settings. The Macintosh computer was developed as a user friendly computer in the mid-1980s, and Apple again had revolutionized the computer industry by developing a system that enable the user to make commands by using a mouse and pull-down menu schema that bypassed the need to learn the more traditional keyboard commands for initiating computer functions.

Within the health care setting, "the first patient monitoring system was implemented at the National Institute of Health Clinic in Maryland" in 1961[5] during the first phase of medical computing-experimentation.[5](p35) Computers emerged in clinical laboratory settings in the 1960s (second phase of medical computing-processing of medical data)[5](p36) and have continued to grow in sophistication in this area. In 1968, "a 19-member Automated Laboratory Systems Committee, [composed] of pathologists and chief administrative technologists from Minnesota Hospitals, joined forces with the Minnesota Hospital Services Association's staff to define the objectives of a computerized automated laboratory."[6] In these early days, the laboratory computer was defined primarily as a tool to increase accuracy and to reduce response time. Along the way, however, the computerization of the laboratory has affected the practice of medicine significantly. "In the past, laboratory studies were 'ancillary' —they were a source of information that supplemented the history and physical examination. Now these tests have become increasingly sophisticated, accurate, inexpensive, and available. The information from these sources is rapidly becoming the most useful data for diagnostic evaluation."[7](p132-133) "Just two or three decades ago, a diagnosis was deduced primarily from the patient's history, observations of physiologic status, and any minute pathologic anatomic changes apparent to the naked eye."[8](p 93) Other medical specialties were to follow the laboratory quickly during the third and current phase of medical computing —supporting the information requirements of medicine.[5](p36) A partial listing of computerized medical advances developed by Solomon includes the following:

1. Programmed history-taking.
2. Electrocardiography (including Holter monitoring, computerized exercise testing, and programmable pacemakers)
3. Vectrocardiography.
4. Body surface isopotential maps.
5. Electroencephalography.
6. Pulmonary function tests.
7. Computed medical imaging.
8. Diagnostic ultrasound.
9. Physiologic monitoring (particularly in intensive and coronary care units).
10. Obstetrical and Neonatal Monitoring.
11. Sleep Monitoring[7](p127-225).

In some cases, use of high technology in physical therapy has kept pace with the use of high technology in education, science, and practice within the health science professions, but in many areas it has not. This chapter will be devoted to a discussion of the use of computers in physical therapy research, education, and practice (management and patient care).

Research

The first job of the computer was as a research tool; it now is so entrenched in this role that many research activities will never be attempted without it again.[9] Research in physical therapy spans a continuum from qualitative (participant observation, case studies) to quantitative (double-blind, case-controlled, experimental) studies. The computer is a critical tool in the acquisition, storage, and assessment of data within all of these research methodologies.

Qualitative evaluation demands the collection of in-depth information from the investigator's observations. This kind of data was collected in the past as handwritten (typed) field notes by physical therapy investigators such as Rosemary Scully, EdD, PT. Dr. Scully's doctoral dissertation presented a grounded theory approach to describing the functions of clinical teachers in physical therapy.[11] As Dr. Scully describes it, grounded theory "involves generating theory rather than verifying it. With this approach, the investigator goes into the field free of predetermined theoretical constraints."[11](p7) To generate theory, the observer must record everything that is encountered in the field with as much objectivity as possible. Dr. Scully describes her process of collecting data: "field notes of the observations and conversations were recorded, in rough form, by the investigator in a small notebook she carried with her in the field. After each day in the field, a more complete text of the data was typed at home."[11](p50) With the invention of the transistor, dictating or other audio taping equipment became usable tools in the field (clinic) and provided the investigator with more complete records of observations. For example, Pamela Stanton, EdD, PT, conducted her doctoral dissertation research on mentoring in physical therapy (based on grounded theory) by tape recording interviews while also taking field notes.[12] Audiotapes reduce the time otherwise used to write out field notes and provide a backup for recollections, but they also omit important visual cues of which the investigator must keep in-depth notes. The author found that three modes of recording observations were necessary in studying children with arthritis in a summer camp environment.[13] Detailed field notes, audiotapes, and videotapes all were used to collect information. Traditionally, these field notes, audiotapes, and videotapes then are transcribed by a support person and the investigator codes the notes according to specific pieces of information that emerge from the observations. The notes then are used manually to complete multiple analyses of the data. The first use of computers in this field involved the key punching of a MAG card with each code and then the hand sorting of the data according to the question being studied. Recently, QUAL-LOG, a program for the microcomputer designed to store, code and analyze qualitative data was developed at State University of New York at Buffalo[14] and is greatly enhancing an evaluator's ability to code and sort qualitative data with speed and accuracy. In the future, voice-activated, hand-held microcomputers will make it possible to increase even further the speed with which information is recorded so that the analysis of the data can proceed in a timely fashion. The great advantage then will be to publish the information gained from such studies within a reasonable amount of time. In the future, these techniques can aid greatly in developing an approach to programmed history taking or evaluation of patients' adherence to physical therapy programs.

Computers always have played a key role in the storage and analysis of quantitative data using computer languages such as FORTRAN, BASIC, and COBOL. Recent advancements in this area have been the emergence of microcomputers and programs such as EPI-LOG, D-BASE, and STAT-PAL that provide an investigator with tools that replicate the traditional main frame quantitative-data management packages (eg, SPSS®, SAS®). The quantitative researcher seldom computes statistical equations by hand, slide rule, or calculator, but increasingly relies on software programs to perform these functions. This is not meant to suggest that the quantitative researcher no longer needs to acquire the skills of computing such data. Computers are remarkable in many ways, but they still are only as accurate as the people who program them; even large main frames are subject to error. Major problems still exist with microcomputer hardware and software when large data sets require sophisticated management, and the informed investigator is in the best position to catch errors in such programs based on his expectations of output. At this time, it appears that physical therapy researchers still are relying on main frame computers to store and analyze data, but many are making the change to the microcomputer as the statistical packages become more sophisticated and as the microcomputer memory increases to allow the storage of large data sets.

Until recently, physical therapy clinical researchers relied on imprecise instruments to measure outcomes. In many instances, the techniques allowed for a large margin of error because of the human factor involved in the technique. For example, measuring joint angles with a traditional goniometer when changes in that angle were meant to reflect success or failure of an intervention significantly flawed the research. The advent of the electronic goniometer at University of California at Los Angeles and the continuing development of that technology by Helen J. Hislop, PhD, PT, and her colleagues has begun to bridge the gap between low and high technology and between speculative and precise data. Once the electronic goniometer is perfected, it will lay the groundwork for total limb goniometry during movement and the precise description of joint ranges in normal subjects during normal activities. When such information is available and is programmed, then it will be possible to quantify movement precisely and determine the degree of disability of any one or set of joints during specific functions. The analysis occurring over multiple joints going through multiple cycles will best be accomplished by the user of a computer. Leo Petrowski, MD, of San Diego, is leading the way in understanding the role of the computer in enhancing human movement through his work in paraplegia. Dr. Petrowski uses the computer to provide motor impulses to the lower extremities at the normal speed, duration, and sequence to produce aided ambulation.

Additional groundwork was established by the motion studies conducted by M. Pat Murray, PhD, PT, and physical therapy researchers who are carrying on her work in the study of human gait and motion. This is an area in which computer technology is becoming an integral part of the research process in physical therapy and has already made significant contributions in motion studies of professional and olympic athletes. In these instances, the computer is being used to collect, store, and analyze data.

Many improved data acquisition tools are becoming available to physical therapy evaluators. For example, computerized exercise equipment quantifies output and provides a record of that output and computerized electromyographic equipment gives more accurate information through printouts of individual motor unit output or summated potentials.

Physical therapy research data can be stored on main frame computers, but it can also be stored using microcomputer file systems which are available in a variety of programs. In the future, such data could be stored for maximal usefulness in a physical therapy database either at the facility, state, regional, or national level using telecommunications linkages. In 1986, the Board of

Directors of the APTA voted to fund the establishment of a national database and issued a Request for Proposal to nationally recognized individuals and organizations to design the system and establish the mechanism for the collection and maintenance of the data. This action was critical because it represented the commitment of the Association to invest resources in establishing the mechanism for ongoing research within the profession without relying on other health statistic agencies' good will to make the data available in a form usable to the Association or to the individual researcher.

Perhaps the greatest challenge facing physical therapy research in which high technology is used maximally by the individual researcher and by collectives of researchers is the need to develop a standard nomenclature for the profession. Such standardization will be necessary for the storage and retrieval of information. If, for instance, we come to believe, as Lawrence Weed, MD, University of Vermont, has advocated in the development of the Problem Oriented Medical Record (POMR), that the medical record is the central point for collection, storage, and analysis of patient information, then it will be critical that all physical therapists use the same name for variables such as disease, disability, or movement if we hope to use the record as a future source of data.

Education

"The rapid growth of electronic technology in the past two decades presents universities with the first major transformation in the transmission and storage of ideas and information since the introduction of printing in fifteenth-century Italy and Germany. It is an absolutely shattering development, requiring rethinking for nearly every aspect of higher education."[15] We are on the verge of this technology emerging as a new academic tool for all students. "The function of the University is to engage in teaching and research of the highest attainable quality."[16] Teaching can be enhanced by developing the computer as a teaching tool to the same extent that it has been developed as a research tool.[17] Public schools are encouraging students to use computers in the classroom and computerization of the classroom is one of the major research agendas for public schools.[18] The computer is being used in a number of ways within education. It is a common fact that students learn at different paces and the classroom teacher has often become frustrated trying to accommodate those different paces in such a way that the faster learner does not get bored and the slower learner does not become overwhelmed. Computer assisted instruction provides one of the answers to this dilemma by allowing student/teacher pacing of the material. The emergence of the microcomputer on college campuses is predicted to change the manner in which students in a higher education setting are taught and the manner in which they learn.[17]

Computers have become an integral part of several university programs (engineering, math, business) and in several instances universities (Dartmouth, Massachusetts Institute of Technology, Carnegie-Mellon) have taken on the characteristics of a computer-intensive campus in that they adopt computer literacy as a prerequisite of an undergraduate program and they encourage or require all students to purchase a personal computer upon admission to the University. Computer literacy means that the students learn to use the computer in their daily work as students so that they have an equal opportunity to pursue careers in business, engineering, or math and to compete in the marketplace that is becoming increasingly dominated by the use of high technology. In addition, these campuses also display other characteristics such as having local area networks, computerized library collections, on-line campus-wide bulletin boards, conversions of campus newspapers to on-line bulletin boards, and a growing number of professors who convert classroom hand outs to the computer to be down-loaded by the student.19 Such campus-wide changes are expected to bring about changes in teaching and learning.

In his doctoral dissertation, Dale Chapman sought "to predict the effects which microcomputer technology is likely to have on undergraduate instruction within the next twenty years. A forcasting technique known as the Delphi method [was] used to collect data from experts representing America's major computer hardware companies, software companies, colleges and universities, and computer consultant organizations.[20]

Among the predictions that resulted from his study, Chapman states the following:

1. The microcomputer will open the door for more remote electronic coursework from homes, offices, dorms, and remote workstations but will not diminish the need for a physical campus, for personal interaction with the faculty, or for traditional student services.
2. Over the next twenty years, microcomputer technology will create more student demand for personal interaction with faculty members and traditional student services and will free faculty members and students from much of the drudgery of teaching-learning, permitting more and "higher quality" student-faculty personal interaction.
3. The role of the faculty will not change as a result of microcomputer technology.
4. Within the next twenty years, multicontextual learning environments will predominate in undergraduate education. Laboratories, for example, will change significantly as students spend more hours in "virtual labs" doing computer laboratory simulations than in actual labs conducting actual experiments.
5. Faculty members will continue to control curriculum and retain traditional roles as teachers and researchers through the year 2005.
    a. Teachers will function in the higher domains of learning-analysis and synthesis —while the computers certify learning in the lower domains.
    b. Faculty members will take on more of a facilitator-mentor role.
    c. Faculty members will be seen as resource people.
    d. The organization of instruction will change away from traditional departmental divisions toward some new organizational configuration (eg, knowledge-based centers).

e. Faculty members will have to be prepared more adequately in computer applications in education.

f. Microcomputer networking in the year 2005 will create a "permanent" group of lifelong learners who upon graduation will continue to communicate electronically with faculty members, thus stretching out their education.

g. Faculty members from all discipline areas of undergraduate instruction are likely to feel the effects of the technology within the next twenty years.

6. It seems likely that in the next twenty years microcomputer technology will increase student access, individualization of instruction and differentiation between institutional types.[20]

Chapman summarizes these predictions in the following statements:

1. The quality of educational technology and speed at which it is created will determine the extent to which microcomputer technology revolutionizes undergraduate instruction over the next twenty years.

2. Microcomputer technology will supplement and not supplant traditional undergraduate teaching-learning; however, teaching pedagogy and the traditional teacher-student relationship will alter radically.

3. Microcomputer technology will increase efficiency in teaching and learning, thereby decreasing the number of years required to complete undergraduate degree or thereby raising the quality and quantity of what is taught-learned in a traditional four-year degree program.[20]

As Chapman points out, the considerable data available regarding change has demonstrated that the resistance to change at the university level is greater than at any level of schooling.[20,21] Physical therapy education, however, is undergoing a major transition as it shifts to a postbaccalaureate degree program and is making significant curricula change to prepare the physical therapist of the twenty-first century. Many physical therapy educators see this time of change as a time of opportunity. It has been postulated that "the greater the extent to which microcomputers become both a cultural and a work-tool technology, the greater will be the demand and need for their use in schools."[21] The extent to which physical therapy practice and research uses the microcomputer no doubt will drive the extent to which this technology is used within the educational environment. It is apparent from the publications of physical therapy researchers and clinicians in areas such as workplace ergonomics, biomedical engineering for the handicapped, and analyses of productivity, that high technology is becoming more important to physical therapy practice and research. Many physical therapy educators therefore are moving to form new alliances with computer education, business, engineering, and math departments as they plan postbaccalaureate degree programs.

The triple challenge here is for physical therapy educators:

1. to introduce computer literacy as a prerequisite for obtaining a degree in physical therapy in order to prepare physical therapists adequately to bridge the gap between a highly technical society and the profession of physical therapy;

2. to model the use of the computer in faculty member (academic and clinical) research activities and expect its use in student research activities; and
3. to teach the use of the computer in practice management, clinical research, patient care, and lifelong learning.

Practice Management

The primary use of computers in practice has been focused on practice management and information management. In a recent survey of computer use in 550 physical therapy practices in Missouri, Illinois and Indiana, Gogia and Braatz further described computer use in physical therapy.[22] The investigators went on to conduct a national survey in *Clinical Management in Physical Therapy*, a nonreferred magazine of the APTA. A second survey yielded 494 respondents from a distribution of that magazine to over 36,000 physical therapists, yielding a response rate of just over 1%.[23] Because the first study yielded a 65% response rate, I have greater confidence in the first survey in which "72% of the respondents were using the computer for entering charges on the hospital system; 65% were using it for recording patient charges; 59% were using it to receive physicians' orders directly from the ward; 38% for patient billing; 33% for patient records; 21% for Cybex data reduction and interpretation of results; 19% for productivity monitoring; 19% for word processing; 16% for practice analysis and management reporting; 14% for telecommunication; 11% for quality assurance activities; and 1% in each of the following: accounts receivable, accounts payable, budgeting, insurance claim processing and electronic mail service."[22]

As this study points out, the majority of respondents who use computers in their practice use practice management applications that fall into three general categories: financial accounting systems, word processing, and information services.

In the area of practice management, the use of the computer by physical therapists seems to have followed the technological advances in business administration, and in many cases physical therapists have brought computer management techniques into physical therapy office settings (both institutionally based and private) at a high degree of sophistication.

Financial Accounting Systems

Physical therapists in institutional or private practice settings are installing a variety of computers in their practices. In some instances, physical therapists are tying directly into the institutional main frame in the accounting area and having all of the therapists input daily charges; in other situations, therapists are installing computers within their practice environments ranging from microcomputers to large memory capacity computers.

A national survey conducted by the American Hospital Association in 1962 revealed that only 39 hospitals were using computers. By 1976, that number had increased to 3,983 hospitals that either leased or owned computers.[24](p9-11) These computers formed the core of the hospital information systems (HIS) that provided hospital wide capabilities to facilitate day-to--day operation. Among the characteristics of hospital information systems today, there are on-line terminals 1) to transmit information from the admitting area to the financial system regarding admissions, discharges and transfers (ADT) and 2) to communicate from the nurses stations to such areas as laboratories, pharmacy, admitting, and physical therapy. Charges are collected as a by-product of this communication system.[24](p9-11) In some institutions of which the Texas Institute of Research and Rehabilitation probably is the premier example, the entire institution is computerized with central reporting directed to the nursing unit through the patient's chart. In such a system, the patient's day is managed in such a way that meals are not missed, time is not lost by two departments scheduling the patient at the same time, and there is increased efficiency of care and reporting among team members.

Once the practice manager or budget office has set up the appropriate spread sheets and installed a program to manipulate specific information, daily ledgers can be maintained by the therapists or the support staff responsible for recording charges. Many financial systems will produce a bill automatically at a specified interval; prepare the bill for mailing, including filling out the appropriate insurance form; and indicate the billing status instantaneously for all of the practice's patients while it not only maintains the practice's inventory, tax information, and productivity statistics but prints out any of this information in presentation form (charts, graphs) at any point in time.

Depending on the hardware available in the practice, a variety of business software packages can be used to manage the financial affairs of the practice. Among the most commonly used packages today is Lotus1,2,3. This program can be purchased in a spread sheet-based application or a word processing-based application.

Because of some of the unique practice situations that may involve multiple cost-centers within for-profit and not-for-profit ventures, many physical therapists are customizing their financial management systems by consulting with business application programmers who tailor the software to the needs of the individual practices. Some physical therapists who have purchased such consulting services have found the end product consistently useful in solving unexpected problems. One of the reasons for the level of satisfaction certainly could be the software, but additional advantages seem to be related to the continuation of the consulting service for problem solving and for the ongoing training of one person —usually the office manager —to remain current in this particular aspect of the practice. The ultimate goal of many of these practices is to be able to exchange information using telecommunications networks in transmitting the most current information available regarding the financial health of the practice within a financial network that may include 1) for the private practitioner, bankers, accountants, tax advisors, boards of directors, and distant offices, and 2) for the institutionally based physical therapist, the financial administrator, the operations administrator, the appropriate department-based personnel, the accounting department, the budget director and other members of the financial management team.

Word Processing and Information Services

"Word processing involves three components: people, machines and procedures" that come together to improve written communications.[25] The office of the 1980s is an office in which the secretarial role has changed from that of a transcriptionist-receptionist whose primary responsibility in a physical therapy practice was to type patient-related correspondence, evaluations, and progress notes to that of a person who not only maintains basic secretarial skills but is called on increasingly to transfer those skills to computer hardware and software. Word processors used to be considered nothing more than enhanced typewriters. They allowed the operator to establish a format for the documents, kern words to justify margins, cut and paste portions of the document, retrieve portions of the document from other files, merge names and addresses for more efficient mailing, and automatically check spelling and word usage. With the development of desktop publishing, however, word processing has taken on many new dimensions including screening portions of the documents, setting columns, controlling type more precisely and providing a feeling of using a layout environment similar to a typesetting operation as opposed to working in a typewriter environment.[26] Such a system now makes it possible for those in a clinical practice to produce patient newsletters, patient education materials, and public education materials, and generally, to increase the flow of information without incurring significant cost.

First-generation patient education products now are available for use directly on the computer to teach specific exercises, with demonstrations and to develop spread sheets to record progress.[27] Such programs no doubt will develop into sophisticated software in which physical therapists will give a patient education prescription to the office personnel and receive an individualized patient education packet, complete with graphics, in minutes.

The secretarial area is becoming more sophisticated in its ability to communicate directly with other offices, departments, and patient units forming local area networks. Physical therapy secretarial areas contain computer work stations for each office worker, with additional work stations for the professional staff, students, or part-time employees; they additionally center an ample number of modems for those department functions carried on over telecommunications networks. Such systems are expensive to set up. As a matter of fact, "information processing accounts for as much as 23%-29% of the health care cost for hospitalized patients (Richart, 1976)."[8](p6) Several business researchers have developed mechanisms for determining the short-term and long-term cost-benefit of computerized information systems in hospitals.

The nature of office work also is changing. Secretaries may be asked to type from dictation, but they are asked increasingly to put the text into an appropriate software program and then format the finished product. For instance, an office newsletter may be produced using such variables as multiple columns, special messages, regular features, and running headers. The secretary inputs typed material using one of many desktop publishing software packages.

Many secretaries find that they are asked to rework material as many as four times more often than they were asked in the past. As a reviewer of grants, I have found that the quality of the writing in grant proposals and the physical presentation of the proposal has changed significantly over the past several years; I attribute many of those changes to the improved word processing services now available to the researcher.

In some cases, increased familiarity with word processing by individual department members is reducing the number of office staff where staff were employed strictly as transcriptionists. These reductions will increase as the technology advances toward voice-activated systems. Such systems will allow the therapists to call in notes or transfer dictation from the tape recorders to the computer and receive the text in rough form. The secretary then will format the edited text. This process will cut down significantly on the time from a visit to the finished piece of correspondence, evaluation report, or progress note. Office staff who are able to make the transition to the high technology office are offering new and expanded services and are changing the perceptions of the role of office staff as they advance the department's level of sophistication in office computer functions.

In addition to written office-based communications, many institutions are moving toward computerized patient records and centralized storage and retrieval systems. At Duke University, for example, Total Medical Record (TMR) has been developed to manage a patient's encounter from the time an appointment is made to the closing of the patient's account.[7](p237) Another system, PROMIS, (Problem-Oriented Medical Information System), is based on an automated problem-oriented medical record to interrelate the patient's history, treatment records, and findings of tests that bear on a specific problem.[7](p238) and COSTAR (Computer-Stored Ambulatory Record System), is a flexible medical and management information system designed by the Massachusetts General Hospital Laboratory of Computer Science between 1968 and 1975 in collaboration with Digital Equipment Corporation, the National Center for Health Services Research, and the Mitre Corporation. It includes registration, medical data, accounts receivable, report-generator, and electronic-mail functions."[7](p239) Many other record systems are emerging now but appear to be derivations of one of the three major systems.

Patient Care

High technology has played an increasing role in the development of upper extremity prostheses for many years. The demand for precise movement has led to significant advances in prosthetics, which now is playing a role in lower extremity prostheses as well. In some of this work, EMG temporal signatures are used to control the prosthesis. "Using preprogrammed mathematical algorithms for one-or two-side temporal EMG signature identification, it [multifunctional controller] allows an amputee to control an above-elbow or shoulder-disarticulation prosthesis via a microcomputer by contracting specific sets of muscles. It similarly allows a partially paralyzed person to activate a powered-brace system by contracting muscles at the vicinity of the paralyzed limb."[28] Some of the leaders in this field have brought this technology from other countries where the cost of such high technological devices was absorbed more easily by the health care systems. As high technology continues to decrease in price and as the consumer continues to demand greater precision, such prosthetic devices will continue to evolve.

Physical therapy practice is influenced significantly by human engineering (ergonomics), which "deals with designing mechanized devices for efficient use by human beings."[29] This application is most obvious in the rehabilitation center setting where function is enhanced greatly by the communication and mobility devices developed for patients with severe motor impairments. A growing area of interest to the physical therapist is appropriate seating for patients who must engage in a variety of work and recreational tasks. This area and the whole field of work-capacity evaluation has a great potential for using computers to evaluate the dynamics of sitting and working.

In some cases, high technology devices such as the electronic goniometer make their way gradually from the research laboratory to practice. In other instances, however, exercise equipment simultaneously reaches the practice and the research markets. For instance, The Cybex was developed originally as a research tool with the anticipation that it eventually would become a practice tool. The demand from practice was so great for this device that it has become both a practice and a research tool.

Other exercise equipment has come from the cardiology field. Computerized ergometers and treadmills were developed originally for use in the stress testing area. Again, the demand from physical therapy practice has been so great that these and other cardiovascular conditioning pieces of equipment (eg, Life-Cycle, computerized step-test) are being used in both practice and research.

The message being transmitted to the researchers is that practice demands more objective, precise equipment that can be used to evaluate and to treat individuals while storing the information for use at a later time, either in evaluating that same patient again or in performing a retrospective analysis of the patient sample.

In addition to the use of information management systems in the exercise and adaptive equipment areas, physical therapists are using the concepts of clinical decision analysis in determining the outcome of treatment choices. First adapted by the clinical laboratory from mathematics and engineering, clinical decision making algorithms are being used in medicine to determine the value of selecting specific tests to determine diagnoses and to predict prognosis if specific treatment regimens are selected. The technology to develop such algorithms is being made available on microcomputers, but it is still in the early stages of that development. This innovation can play a significant role in teaching physical therapy students, making clinical decisions, and determining the high priorities for clinical research. The models can be built using expert experience, but the more proven the information at each decision node, the greater the confidence in the outcome. This technological advance can turn the intuitive judgment of the experienced clinicians into a logical series of decisions and make clinical decision making a process that can be learned and applied by clinicians regardless of their experience with a particular clinical problem. Such an advance will not only affect the practice of physical therapy greatly but the areas of education and research as well.

Ethical Considerations

One of the concerns that faces an evolving highly technical society is that of "high tech" versus high touch.[30] In a profession such as physical therapy there is great therapeutic value in touching the patients. There also is an ever-increasing number of manual skills physical therapists must not lose. The depersonalization of the computerized physical therapy practice must be balanced by a humanizing element within practice. The ethical concerns that will evolve from computerization must be on the research agenda for physical therapy in the next decade. A brief review of the literature in education related to the computerization of the campus suggests that issues such as confidentiality, privacy, and equal opportunity will emerge as more campuses emerge as computer-intensive.[19] Other interesting and less obvious concerns must be addressed such as the shift in research emphasis toward those areas that can be studied more easily and completely using high technology.

Business is dealing with computer crime issues related to the unauthorized copying of software and the pirating of business innovations by breaking computer passwords. These indeed are crimes, and there is a legal recourse in solving these problems. The issue of privacy, however, is not as clearly defined. The Privacy Act of 1974 laid legal groundwork for protecting privacy but did not anticipate the growth of computers and the possible exploitation of the public through the indiscriminate collection of personal information that then would be accessible. The protection of privacy and the needs of a technologically advanced society to have access to that information I believe is the predominant ethical issue we are facing in terms of information management.

Role of APTA

At this time, the APTA has not developed a plan detailing its role in advancing high technology in physical therapy. As an organizational entity primarily responsible for the management of information, it is moving toward a more highly technical operation. In 1985, the Board of Directors adopted Detailed Program Descriptions (DPDs) that began the process of developing a telecommunication network between APTA and its components. In 1986, the Board also adopted a DPD that would allow APTA staff to investigate the use of image management (videodiscs) in the storage of the Association's archieves. Currently, the publications of the Association have articles related to computer use and the Journal has recently installed a Computer Column.

The APTA certainly has many options available regarding the role it will play in high technology. At one end of the spectrum it can continue its current level of activity in the area, anticipating that as societal demands change, the profession will meet the demand. However, I believe that the APTA has an opportunity to provide a significant service to its members by actively promoting the use of high technology in physical therapy. Among the many activities the Association may undertake in the future, I propose the following:

1. Name a task force to develop a white paper on information management in physical therapy.

2. Continue to develop a national database and expand it in such a way that individuals can add to the data and can analyze the data using standard software such as SPSS or SAS.

3. Develop a computer-based information system for APTA that will cut across all APTA departments and components.

4. Establish an APTA program for monitoring computer applications in practice, research, and education.

5. Establish a physical therapy computer service center to scan the computer market and publish hardware and software information related to physical therapy applications and to produce physical therapy software.

6. Develop mechanisms to communicate to the membership and the public regarding high technology in physical therapy.

7. Support educational programs in information management in physical therapy.

8. Appoint a task force or commission a group to establish standardized nomenclature in physical therapy.

References

1. Beninger J: Information society and the control revolution. Computer-World, November 3, 1986, p 147.
2. Cougar JD: New books aid managers in organizing information systems. ComputerWorld, June 23, 1986, p 87.
3. The computer age. ComputerWorld, November 3, 1986, p 15.
4. Baldridge JV, Roberts JW, Weiner TA: The Campus and the microcomputer revolution. New York, NY, Macmillan Publishing Co, 1984.
5. Blum BI: Clinical information systems. New York, NY, Springer-Verlag Inc, New York, 1986, p 35-36.
6. Westlake GE, Bennington JL: Automation and Management in the Clinical Laboratory, p 205, University Park Press, Baltimore, MD, 1972.
7. Solomon M: Using Computers in The Practice of Medicine. Englewood Cliffs, NJ, Prentice Hall Inc, 1985, p 127-239.
8. Bronzino JD: Computer Applications for Patient Care. Reading, MA, Addison-Wesley Publishing Co, 1982, p 6, 93.
9. Mosmann C: Academic Computers in Service. San Francisco, CA, Jossey-Bass Inc, Publishers, 1973, p 2.
10. Bogdan RC, Biklen SK: Qualitative Research for Education. Boston, MA, Allyn & Bacon Inc, 1982.
11. Scully R: Clinical Teaching of Physical Therapy Students in Clinical Education. Doctoral Dissertation. Ann Arbor, MI, University of Microfilms, 1974.

12. Stanton P: Mentoring Relationships in Physical Therapy. Doctoral Dissertation. Ann Arbor, MI, University Microfilms, 1984.
13. Walter J: Developing a Camp for Children with Arthritis, Preliminary Data of Study in Progress. Hanover, NH, Dartmouth-Hitchcock Arthritis Center, 1986.
14. Bogdan RC: Qualitative Evaluation, University of Vermont, Burlington, VT, Summer, 1984.
15. Keller G: Academic Strategy. Baltimore, MD, The Johns Hopkins University Press, 1983, p 19.
16. Bok D: Beyond The Ivory Tower. Cambridge, MA, Harvard University Press, 1982, p 18.
17. Bok D: Higher Learning. Cambridge, MA, Harvard University Press, 1986.
18. Lazerson M, McLoughlin JB, McPherson B, et al: An Education of Value. New York, NY, Cambridge University Press, 1986.
19. Walter J: Ethical Dilemmas of Computerizing the College Campus. Doctoral dissertation, Ann Arbor, MI, University Microfilms, 1989.
20. Chapman D: The Effects of Microcomputer Technology on Undergraduate Instruction: A Delphi Forecast. Doctoral Dissertation: Ann Arbor, MI, University Microfilms, 1987.
21. Pogrow S: Education in the Computer Age. Sage Publications Inc, Newbury Park, CA, 1983.
22. Gogia PP, Braatz JH: Computers applications in physical therapy practice: Results of the 1986 CM Survey. Clinical Management in Physical Therapy 7(1): 18-20, 1987.
23. Gogia PP, Braatz JH Computer applications in physical therapy practice: Results of the 1986 CM survey. Clinical Management in Physical Therapy. 7(1):18-20, 1987.
24. Zielstorff RD: Computers in Nursing. p. 9-11, Nursing Resources, Wakefield, MA, 1980.
25. Norris DE, Skilbeck CE, Hayward AE, et al: Microcomputers in Clinical Practice. New York, NY, John Wiley & Sons Inc, 1985, p 63.
26. Farber D: Writing your own ticket. MACWORLD. PCW Communications, December 1986, p 100.
27. MacMuscle. Software package. Tech 2000. 263 Lagonia Street, Newport Beach, CA, 92663, 1984.
28. Eden HS, Eden M: Microcomputers in Patient Care. Park Ridge, NJ, Noyes Publications, 1981, p 183.
29. Covvey DH, Craven NH, McAlister NH: Concepts and Issues in Health Care Computing. St. Louis, MO, CV Mosby Co, 1985, p 136.
30. Naisbitt J: Megatrends. New York, NY, Warner Books Inc, 1982.

Bibliography
Baldridge, JV, Roberts, JW and Weiner, TA. The Campus and The Microcomputer Revolution. Macmillan Publishing Co. New York. 1984.
Beninger, J. "Information Society and The Control Revolution." ComputerWorld. November 3, 1986.

Blum, BI. Clinical Information Systems. Springer-Verlag Pubs. New York, NY. 1986.

Bogdan, RC and Biklen, SK. Qualitative Research for Education. Allyn and Bacon, Inc.. Boston, MA. 1982.

Bok, D. Beyond The Ivory Tower. Harvard University Press. Cambridge, MA. 1982.

Bok, D. Higher Learning. Harvard University Press, Cambridge, MA. 1986.

Bronzino, JD. Computer Applications for Patient Care. Addison-Wesley Publishing Co. Reading, MA. 1982.

Carson, ER, Cramp, DG, eds. Computers and Control in Clinical Medicine. Plenum Press. New York, NY. 1985.

Chapman, D. The Effects of Microcomputer Technology On Undergraduate Instruction: A Delphi Forecast. Graduate School of Education of Harvard University. University Microfilms. Ann Arbor, MI.

Cougar, JD. "New Books Aid Managers in Organizing Information Systems." ComputerWorld. June 23, 1986.

Covvey, DH, Craven, NH, McAlister, NH. Concepts and Issues in Health Care Computing. CV Mosby Co. St. Louis, MO. 1985.

Eden, HS, Eden, M. Microcomputers in Patient Care. Noyes Medical Pubs. Park Ridge, NJ. 1981.

Farber, D. "Writing Your Own Ticket. "MACWORLD. PCW Communications, Inc.. 501 Second Street. San Francisco, CA. Dec. 1986.

Flynn, GJ. Medicine in The Age of The Computer. Prentice-Hall, Inc.. Englewood Cliffs, NJ. 1986.

Gogia, PP, Braatz, JH. "Computer Applications in Physical Therapy Practice: Results of The 1986 CM Survey." Clinical Management, Vol. 7, No. 1. American Physical Therapy Association. Alexandria, VA. 1987.

Gogia, PP, Braatz, JH. "Computers and The Physical Therapist: A Survey." Clinical Management, Vol. 6, No. 2. American Physical Therapy Association. Alexandria, VA. 1986.

Hannah, KJ, Guillemin, EJ, Conklin, DN, eds. Nursing Uses of Computers and Information Science. North-Holland Pubs. New York, NY. 1985.

Keller, G. Academic Strategy. The Johns Hopkins University Press. Baltimore, Maryland. 1983.

Lapham, LH, ed. High Technology & Human Freedom. Smithsonian International Symposia Series. Smithsonian Institution Press. Washington, D.C. 1985.

Lazerson, M, McLaughlin, JB, McPherson, B, and Bailey, SK. An Education of Value. Cambridge University Press. New York. 1986.

MacMuscle. Software Package. Tech 2000. 263 Lagonia St. Newport Beach, CA. 1984.

Moreau, R. The Computer Comes of Age. The MIT Press. Cambridge, MA. 1984.

Mosmann, C. Academic Computers in Service. Jossey-Bass Publishers. San Francisco. 1973.

Naisbitt, J. Megatrends. Warner Books, New York. 1982.

Norris, DE, Skilbeck, CE, Hayward, AE, and Torpy, DM. Microcomputers in Clinical Practice. John Wiley & Sons. New York, NY. 1985.

Perrolle, JA. Computers and Social Change: Information, Property and Power. Wadsworth Publishing Co. Belmont, CA. 1987.

Pogrow, S. Education in The Computer Age. Sage Publications. Beverly Hills, CA. 1983. as cited in Chapman.

Ryan, GA and Monroe, KE. Computer Assisted Medical Practice: -The AMA's Role. Center for Health Services Research and Development. American Medical Association. Chicago, IL. 1971.

Scholes, M, Bryan, Y, and Barber, B, eds. The Impact of Computers on Nursing: An International Review. North-Holland, Pubs. New York, NY. 1983.

Scully, R. Clinical Teaching of Physical Therapy Students in Clinical Education. University Microfilms. Ann Arbor, MI. 1974.

Solomon, M. Using Computers in The Practice of Medicine. Prentice-Hall, Inc.. Englewood Cliffs, NJ. 1985.

Stanton, P. Dissertation on Mentoring Relationships in Physical Therapy, in publication by University Microfilms. Ann Arbor, MI.

St. Lawrence, K. Computerized Clinical Nursing Reference Information System. Oryn Pubs, Inc. 1985.

Stolurow, LM, Peterson, TI, and Cunningham, AC, eds. Computer Assisted Instruction in The Health Professions. Entelek Inc.. Newburyport, MA. 1970.

"The Computer Age." Computerworld. November 3, 1986.

Walter, J. Research in progress. "Experiential Learning Project for Children with Arthritis. Dartmouth-Hitchcock Arthritis Center. Hanover, NH. 1985-present.

Walter, J. Dissertation. Ethical Dilemmas of Computerizing The College Campus: A Delphi Study. 1987.

Westlake, GE, and Bennington, JL. Automation and Management in The Clinical Laboratory. University Park Press. Baltimore, MD. 1972.

Zielstorff, RD, ed. Computers in Nursing. Nursing Resources. Wakefield, MA. 1980.

CHAPTER 11

Interdisciplinary Practice: An Opportunity for Leadership

Patricia Gillespie, MPH, PT
Polly Fitz, MA, RD
Carol Gordon, PhD, PT

Introduction

The value of interdisciplinary activities clearly emerges when complex problems arise—when many points of view are used to broaden the perspectives and when many technical areas of expertise are required for the specific tasks. Historically, like many other social experiments, collaborative structures have had limited stability. The enduring quality of these structures has largely been dependent on the commitment and the relationships of those involved, the strong leadership skills in all members, and a supportive environment. Until recently in American industry, the expertise and power of collaborative structures has been overlooked. However, with continual changes in the health care system, models need to be developed that will fit any contingency. One organizational approach used in a changing environment is the collaborative model.

In this chapter on interdisciplinary practice, collaboration is defined as the professional activity of two or more health professionals with a common task or goal. The characteristics of this interdisciplinary process may be seen on a continuum from a multidisciplinary arrangement where members of each discipline function independently to an interdependent relationship which may transcend the individual behaviors of each discipline. The discussion will include the social, economic, and political implications for interdisciplinary practice for physical therapy.

Interdisciplinary Practice

Interdisciplinary practice is based on the premise that the functional requirements for the tasks or work to be performed are best accomplished by a collection of competencies or skills needed for a desired result not possible with one discipline. The assumption is that a synergistic effect is achieved when expertise is pooled and directed toward health care problem-solving. The analysis of the health care work of both the diagnostic and therapeutic tasks performed by the involved disciplines will clearly indicate the characteristics of that interdependence. This interdependence may occur concurrently, sequentially, or serially.[1]

Collaboration

The interaction required between disciplines in an interdependent relationship will necessitate some degree of collaboration. One view of collaboration is described as a contractual relationship between the health professionals and between the health professionals and the client. The relationship may be:

the "referral'" when one practitioner refers the client/patient to another for service and a new contract is established;

the relationship may be a "consultation" when two or more Practitioners discuss the diagnosis or treatment of a client but retain the original contract with the primary practitioner;

the collegial or team relationship when the client interacts with all practitioners either directly or indirectly and may even be a part of the process. In the latter case, the contract is with the group or with a subset of the practitioners.

Clearly in all cases, multiple disciplines are involved: sequential process in the first, concurrent in the second, and perhaps serially in the collegial or group situation.[2]

Collaboration requires highly developed communication and group process skills. The literature of health team development points out the need for the application of the principles and theories of organizational development with particular reference to skills in collaboration. The required competencies for collaboration are to clarify the expectations of the "agreements" in the relationships, to agree on the decision-making processes, and to maintain an open climate for problem-solving. In the collegial or team situation, the process is a negotiation of the relationships which includes establishing agreed-upon goals, defining the necessary required expertise and roles, and determining the decision-making processes to be used. It accepts the premise that change and renegotiation can take place at any time.[3]

The Organization of Interdisciplinary Practice

An interdisciplinary practice may be a formal structural entity, stable, certain, and an integral part of a larger organizational framework. These groups or "teams" usually have a clear purpose, clear membership in terms of disciplines, and explicit processes of decision-making. These teams can be utilized either on demand or full time depending on the tasks. They are task focused and exist primarily because the purposes could not be met independently. The tasks are interdependent at some point, either reciprocally, serially, or in some other structural configuration. Expectations are usually explicit and communication patterns are clear. Examples in rehabilitation are the stroke teams, burn teams, pain teams, and, in the school systems, the pupil planning teams.

By contrast, other forms of interdisciplinary practice may not have that formal structure and may function more on a contingency basis. The success of these groups in accomplishing the goals is highly dependent on the negotiating skills and the values of the practitioners. It is also dependent on the support from the system to provide the freedom for the interactive practice to take place. According to Blanchard, independent decision-making is dependent on the situational requirements and on the maturity and the technical level of the individuals. [4] Leadership is shared at all levels of the system.

Interdisciplinary Roots in Health Policy Development

The federal government and private foundations have attempted to stimulate the development of innovative interdisciplinary systems of care over the past two decades. The Office of Economic Opportunity mandated the establishment of Neighborhood Health Centers with primary health care teams in the late 1960's. Team development programs in these centers and in medical schools were supported in large part by grants from the Robert Wood Johnson Foundation.[5]

Somewhat later, interdisciplinary education projects were federally funded. The most notable project was a community based educational program in the College of Allied Health Professions at the University of Kentucky (Kentucky January and later Kentucky May) where interdisciplinary student teams worked on community health problems in rural Kentucky as part of their educational program.[6] The Area Health Education Center projects mandated interdisciplinary involvement as a condition for funding [7] as did the Humanistic Health Care Education grants. The Pediatric Research and Training Centers under the Department of Education, and the associated projects under the University Affiliated Systems program focused on the need for interdisciplinary practice in pediatrics. Public Law 94-142,which includes the need for the provision of health services for special children in the school systems, mandates participation of the disciplines in their Pupil Planning Teams.[8]

More recently, the Geriatric Education Centers, both federally funded and privately supported, mandate interdisciplinary practice in the care of the elderly and in the education of professionals for interdisciplinary practice. The Veterans Administration Interdisciplinary Team Development projects in geriatrics have stimulated education, service, and also have strong evaluation components. Although the projects for the training of personnel in the HIV/AIDS epidemic does not specify an interdisciplinary structure, the implication is evident with the inclusion of all health professionals in the programs developed by the Educational Training Centers.

Interest in the development of interdisciplinary practice is also evident in a group of professionals who have successfully held a series of ten conferences with the purpose of sharing interdisciplinary experiences in both education and practice. Recently, these conferences have given a focus on evaluative research with emphasis on the cost effectiveness of the collaborative models. This informal action group has succeeded in maintaining interest and commitment to an interdisciplinary model for almost two decades.[9]

Need for Interdisciplinary Care

An analysis of the work requirements of a comprehensive and coordinated rehabilitation system clearly indicates that multiple services are needed for most conditions requiring rehabilitation. Almost every diagnosis has indications for a need for improvement in physical, psychological, social, and occupational status. Given the assumption that there are varying degrees of interdependence among professional practitioners to accomplish those objectives, it is further assumed that some degree of an interdisciplinary approach would be required to meet those needs in an organized system to assure quality care.

Certainly, a young woman who has a cerebrovascular accident (CVA) during childbirth and a middle-aged truck driver who has a lumbar laminectomy need multiple rehabilitation services. The woman is in need of physical therapy for mobility, strengthening, transfer and gait training; occupational therapy for Activities of Daily Living training; and perhaps social and psychological services to help hold the family together during this stressful rehabilitation process. With these practitioners working as an interdisciplinary team, priority goals can be reached more efficiently. With the family as active participants in the goal setting process, realistic expectations for the future can be established.

The need for interdisciplinary negotiation skills among rehabilitation personnel is further exemplified in the case of the middle-aged truck driver with the lumbar laminectomy. After palliative physical therapy progressing to strength and mobility work, he will probably be enrolled in a "work hardening" program, a trend in the late 1980's. The negotiation issue emerges between occupational and physical therapy as to the determination of which discipline is most qualified to provide those services. If the work hardening proqram is unsuccessful in the preparation of the client for return to the same work activities, social and vocational services will be needed for job retraining which is an additional issue in negotiation.

The Reality of the Current Environment

The health care environment is experiencing an escalating crisis. The costs of services and goods in the health care industry far outweigh the resources available to meet the high levels of service demands. The rising cost of medical care and the resultant cost control measures have placed a major burden on systems and individuals to provide even basic services. The issue of the determination of basic services is now being debated in Congress and clearly indicates the political nature of the issue.

With a shift in services away from high cost hospital care to new settings, the demands for human resources are increasing in all sectors. The current hospital system is increasingly faced with more complex and severe health problems, with finite resources, with increased regulation, and with both public and private efforts to affect cost containment. With health professionals and health services moving to a less regulated environment to escape the above pressures, the acute care system is experiencing severe problems in meeting societal demands.

Because of limits on the financing of services, a highly competitive environment has emerged. With competition for scarce resources, the political and social forces determine the services to be used. As resources are allocated, the determination of who has access to services is regulated by public policy. Priorities for acute care and primary care have been higher than those for long-term care. However, recent efforts to provide catastrophic insurance and to establish universal basic minimal coverage have been attempts by policymakers to alleviate the disparity in coverage to assure at least a minimum of quality care.

Although some changes have occured to provide for reimbursement of rehabilitation services, these same changes have contributed to the competitive climate in rehabilitation services. For example, in 1988 occupational therapy became reimbursable under part B of the Medicare program. On the one hand, it provided access to those services by the consumer, but it further divided the finite allowances for coverage, creating a competitive environment within the rehabilitation services.

Another example exists within the Health Maintenance Organization financial structure (HM0). The finite dollars from the enrollments are essentially controlled by the primary care physician. The other health personnel then must compete with the physician for a portion of those dollars. The referral process is affected by the value of the services held by the physician.

Economic and political influences clearly play a vital role in determining the participants in the system. Those services eligible for direct payment or, at best, included indirectly in a package fee are more likely to be included. Where there is no reimbursement through insurance or public grants, the inclusion of those services is not likely to occur. Whoever has the power and influence will determine the required service and will control the payment mechanisms. The political element then will influence the process.

Under these conditions, the likelihood of all professionals sharing the pot of resources is dim. If the collaboration, or the multidisciplinary approach can attract business and be reimbursed, it will exist. Even then, there are no guarantees that collaboration will take place. Most of these public mechanisms define services as independent entities. Stimulating or supporting collaboration with financing mechanisms does not exist. Any organizational configuration within a health service institution that builds linkages needs to ensure that each element is reimbursable. Nowhere are there allowances for the time needed to support the collaborative processes involved in integrating the services.

Incentives for professional behavior are often determined by the financial returns to the practitioner and/or the health care organization. This is dependent on the "reimbursable service". This component of the reward system does not foster collaboration. In fact, it supports competition between the providers and the practitioners for the market share of the allowable pool. Although the recent DRG system has attempted to change that process by rewarding the efficient use of an allowable dollar amount for each diagnosis, not for each service used, the behaviors of the professionals are still competitive for that allocated portion of the dollar.

It could be hypothesized that collaboration would be more economical, but there are few studies to support that premise. Evaluative activities from the Veterans Administration project on the geriatric health team programs are beginning to yield some data. [10]

One of the primary reasons that research is minimal on team processes is that productivity measures are related to patient care with no allowances for investigative activities.

Consumer Involvement

Participation on health teams by members of the client system is more a determinant of social norms than of technical requirements. The client/patient, the family, community members, the administrator, clergy, and a host of others in the system of care are included as marginal team members. A new participant in the system is the family caregiver for the older clients. [11] Consumers also need the support of an advocate, particularly with the reimbursement regulations. The case managers have to add this new competency of consultant to the family in addition to the role of coordinating services. Businesses are emerging that offer services to the consumer in following the administrative procedures for receiving reimbursement.

The rise in consumer influence in the selection of services may increase the likelihood of more comprehensive and coordinated systems. In recent years, there has been an increase in the general public awareness of the role of the therapies. That public is the consumer, the patient/client of rehabilitation services. As the consumer becomes more sophisticated, (s)he will demand the most comprehensive and coordinated services possible for the dollar allowances. Active participation of the client in making health care decisions for access to services may require a renewed interest in the service ethic and the need to provide an integrated system of services.

The advent of Preferred Provider Organizations (PPOs) and Health Maintenance Organizations (HMOs) limits consumer choice by putting greater constraints on the free market/free enterprise system by defining the pool of health care givers available for reimbursable services. On the other hand, with increased numbers of practitioners in all of the therapies, the consumer has more choices for care. The options extend beyond the traditional outpatient rehabilitation services of the local hospital. Consumer choice will be based on convenience, quality, and value. Physical therapy has achieved the capacity to provide service in many settings and is in competition with hospital rehabilitation services. In an increasing number of private physical therapy practice settings, multiple services are available. Social service, occupational therapy, nutrition, and speech services are added to attract clients and ensure the market share of the rehabilitation dollar.

Powerful consumer groups such as the American Association for Retired People will also help to influence the quality and availability of care. As the general population ages, their influence and that of other groups will become even more powerful. The rehabilitation professionals may need to collaborate to educate these groups about their services.

Baldwin comments that the hope for interdisciplinary efforts to take hold lies with the public who have clearly stated that they would like to see the quality of their health care enhanced by more realistic and humanistic attitudes and skills.[12] As the public assumes more control over the setting of policy and administration of the health care system, changes will occur. History has provided many powerful examples of this consumer-driven change: interdisciplinary childbirth education programs and provision of health services in the school systems.

Physical Therapy's Search for Status and Independence

The importance of social factors on team membership and participation in interdisciplinary services has been reported extensively. Mentioned frequently are the following: the educational level of the participants; the degree of functional autonomy or interdependence in the tasks to be performed; and the independence as defined by licensure. The presence of a hierarchy within a team structure is largely determined by these factors.

More important, the manifestations of these social norms are evident in the processes used to make decisions, which clearly influence the interdisciplinary process. If independent decision making is valued and is the cultural mode of practice, the likelihood of a collaborative process is diminished. The issues of responsibilty for decisions and liability for dependent practitioners' behaviors tend to place a risk on the process. When all players are equally responsible in the eyes of the courts, team practice is more likely to occur.[13]

Socialization of the health professional places high value on the following: autonomy, expertise, social control of functions, public service, and contributions to the common good. Pellegrino states that to be a professional.."is to make a promise to help, to keep that promise and to do so in the best interest of the patient."[14] The implication is that these service values are prime.

> *Autonomy embodies both the will and action with the individual determining his or her own course of action according to a self designed plan. Autonomy is freedom to govern oneself and make one's own choices according to one's own moral principles based on the central principle that each person is judged to be of intrinsic worth.* Matejski[15]

Therefore, the social development of a group would be affected by its degree of autonomy. Physical therapy has worked long and hard to be recognized as an autonomous profession. First by establishing its own educational standards separate from organized medicine and more recently. by making efforts to amend the practice acts to permit the public to have direct access to physical therapy services. These internal efforts have absorbed the profession for at least two decades. In the efforts to establish autonomy, energy at the organizational level for collaboration and coalition building has been a lower priority, although it still has been present.

Social, developmental theory holds that independence and control over ones destiny is a motivation that precedes the social behaviors of collaboration and task interdependence.[16] If this is the case, the issues surrounding the search for autonomy may have eroded the basic professional ethic for better service at the organizational or macro level.

As stated earlier, it is assumed that a multiplicity of health services are required to meet patient care needs particularly in rehabilitation. Health services must be coordinated and accessible to those in need. However, the physical therapy professional journals are directed to the development of a scientific base for only that area of professional practice independent of any other professional groups. Rarely are contributions cited that are multidisciplinary or related to the impact of the system on patient care outcomes.

On the other hand, the practitioner faced with the problems of providing quality service to the patients/clients is well aware of the interdependence of providers in order to coordinate service delivery. The development of patient care plans requires a battery of diagnostic activities before therapy can proceed. The earlier case clearly indicated needs for social and vocational services in addition to occupational and physical therapy. These contributions are limited only by the organizational and financial constraints that the health care system imposes. The professional values and rewards are still grounded in the achievement of successful or maximal client outcomes.

Who is responsible for insuring the coordination and the adequacy of the services? The independent physical therapy practitioner? The physician or the rehabilitation nurse? Or, is it expected that the expected future level of skill development in physical therapy will negate the necessity of other services? Will the therapist perform all of the multiple functions required for a comprehensive rehabilitation program?

The seeds of a moral dilemma for the individual physical therapist begin to emerge. On the one hand, the profession emphasizes the importance of independence with policies that promote:

1) legal independence from the practice of medicine through the amending of the state licensing practice acts;

2) educational independence through internal standard setting by the profession;

3) an increase in the educational requisite for the entry level to support the above;

4) opposition to physician-owned physical therapy practices;

5) support for direct reimbursement for physical therapy service.

This climate of advocacy for independence sets the values for the professional practitioner. Conversely, it may negate the values for interdependence. It does not acknowledge the realities of those physical therapy practice settings where interdependence and teaming are a norm with quality outcomes.

Meeting Technological Demands

Physical therapy is not unlike many of the health related disciplines where a large increase in the technological development has occured over the past several decades. The population of clients seeking rehabilitation represents those with complex problems requiring not only intensive services from each discipline but extensive and diverse expertise over a long period of time. Rehabilitation nursing, social work, clinical dietetics, occupational therapy, orthotics and prosthetics are only a few of the professions that participate with medicine and physical therapy on the rehabilitation team. Without the expertise of all disciplines, the quality of life for the individuals needing care would be severely jeopardized.

How does the practitioner resolve that dilemma? Can the professions be responsive to the interdependent issues with as much energy as the independent and renew the commitment to service in an environment that requires a collective effort?

Building Teams

The foundations for building teams are found in the concepts of sociotechnical systems design. The concepts have been in organizational theory for almost three decades but only recently applied to health care organizations. [17] The development of "high performing " work systems in industry has emphasized the importance of integration of the technical components of the work and the social elements of the worker.[18]

In breaking down these two elements in high performing teams the social components include, but are not limited to, those factors that influence individual and group behavior: role (expectancy theory); maturation of the individual (Mazlow); group cultural norms and values; and the interactive skills required for participation in problem solving groups.

The principles in sociotechnical systems design include redefining work collectively and acknowledging the incentives for control and self-direction. Power is balanced with the designation of decision making to the appropriate person and work to be done. Boundary spanning and role clarification are included. All of these activities result in increasing the effectiveness of the system.

As yet, there do not appear to be models in the health care delivery system for the resolution of the social and technical dilemmas. It is the basic premise that improved outcomes will be achieved through sociotechnical systems design which supports collaboration. [19] Only a few embrace that philosophy. Until the connection is made that improved outcomes are a result of effective teamwork, health care professionals will not be likely to foster the organization and work redesign.

Education: Preparation for Interdisciplinary Practice

Experience in preparation for interdisciplinary practice was first noted in the Primary Health Team Development projects sponsored by the Robert Wood Johnson Foundation in the ealy 70's. A critical issue that emerged in medical education was the perception that this dimension was somehow additive and placed pressure on an already overburdened educational system. [5]

In discussing the curriculum overload for medical students, Baldwin comments as follows:

From what I have been able to observe, the more pressure applied by the system, the less free in mind and spirit are our students to reflect on knowledge and experience, to explore new ideas and feelings, to experiment with new ways of being with themselves and with others. The learner becomes the teacher of what he has been taught. Is it any wonder that the professional has fallen so far in public esteem?[12]

Such crowding of the curriculum rapidly lends to information overload for the student and increasing isolation and specialization among the teachers themselves.

The rigors and "crunch" of the physical therapy curriculum provide similar comparison to the medical school curriculum. The insular approach to a professional discipline focus in physical therapy education may provide a weak springboard for students as they go out to establish clinical practice with diverse and increasingly frail client systems. In the consumer driven system of the future, the ability to relate with others, such as clients and professionals, will be key in developing successful practice ventures. To become the case manager in new settings will require additional skills and knowledge found in interdisciplinary education; knowledge of other health professional services; knowledge of resources in the system.[20]

The Future

Special attention should be focused on methods of coordinating care in light of current practices. As stated by Williams,

Rapid appearance and expansion of multidisciplinary generic assessment or consultation clinics and services have occured in many settings . . . All the staff disciplines are directly involved with the makeup and planning for the care of patient and family. This development indicates the growing recognition of the team approach.[21]

Significantly, there is a positive correlation between the teams and other caregivers in terms of their colleagiality and their success in managing the care and maintaining and improving the general function level of their patients. The more colleagiality, the more positive the outcomes.[22]

The implications for public policy are primarily directed to the economic incentives. Requiring the interdisciplinary delivery of service or the sharing of resources through the regulations for reimbursement is certainly one approach to facilitate collaborative practice. The interchangeable utilization of disciplines such as the recent "work hardening" programs with occupational and physical therapy involvement includes an interchangeable policy but it is not accepted by either group. Substitution of another health professional or increasing the generic skills may be worrisome to the professional looking at direct reimbursement and independent practice.

It would seem that the imperative is to reaffirm the commitment of the profession to "service", to the contributions to the public good to balance the financial incentives, particularly with the value for quality care as a demand from the consumer. The current model of a multidiscipline practice is primarily based on an economic incentive as a good marketing strategy. Interaction may occur but is not necessarily inherent in the philosophy of practice. Few exceptions exist. Given a reversal of the trend which had limited reimbursed services by Medicare to one that is responsive to the needs of the aged population, collaborative services may begin to flourish.

Achieving independent status and autonomy is a major professional goal. The independent practice model does not explicitly promote collaboration with other disciplines.[23] Some leaders in physical therapy are from the private practice sector. They are the pace setters and are characterized by the independent entrepreneur who aspires to economic and social independence with a medical model. External forces produce conflict and internally, the lack of value for interdisciplinary practice tends to increase the tension and potential conflict. This is reinforced by the educational preparation and early socialization of the professional. However, once physical therapists feel more comfortable with their increased autonomy and independence in practice, perceiving an increase in prestige, collaboration may become more acceptable.

An Action Agenda

The opportunity to be more responsive to the consumer demands and technological requirements requires a commitment to impact on public policy and the organizational responses. [24] The authors would like to suggest the following action agenda for leaders in physical therapy.

For the professional association:

* Clarify the issues of independent practice and interdependent practice.

* Increase the awareness of the value of interdisciplinary practice through publications and presentations at major conferences.

* Establish the priority for interorganizational agreements.

* Promote policies that separate the issues of interdependent practice from reimbursement.

* Establish a priority for the development of organizational liaisons with other health professions.

For the Practitioner:

* Insure that all patient care outcomes meet patient needs.

* Accept the responsibility to develop collaborative models for comprehensive and effective service delivery.

For the Educator:

* Analyze current practices in education in light of the service delivery patterns meeting health care needs.

* Develop learning experiences for both independent and interdependent practice.

* Assume the leadership for setting values for interprofessional behavior.

References

1. Charns M, Schaefer M: Health Care Organizations: A Model for Management. Englewood Cliffs, NJ. Prentice Hall Inc. 1983.
2. Brill N: Teamwork: Working Together in the Human Services. Philadephia, PA. JB Lippincott. 1976.
3. Rubin I, Plovnick M, Fry R: Improving the Coordination of Care: A Program for Health Team Development. Cambridge, MA. Ballinger. 1975.
4. Blanchard K: Situational Leadership Revisited. NTL Managers Handbook. Arlington, VA. NTL Institute. 1983. 73-87.
5. Wise H, Beckhard R, Rubin L, Likyte A: Making Health Teams Work. Cambridge, MA. Ballinger. 1974.
6. Kentucky January Program. Description and Activities, 1974, 1975. Office of Special Programs, College of Allied Health Professions, University of Kentucky, Lexington, KY.
7. The AHEC Bulletin: IV. Winter 1986-87.
8. Brightly B: Training Alliances in Health and Education. A Final Report. Washington DC, American Society of Allied Health Professions. 1986.
9. Cumulative Index of the Proceedings of the Interdisciplinary Health Care Team Conferences 1976-1986 Bowling Green, Ohio. College of Health and Human Services, Bowling Green State University. 1988.
10. Personal communication with Janet Feazell, Veterans Administration, Washington DC.
11. Sheehan N: The Family Care Giver. CARE 1:1 (Fall 1988).
12. Baldwin DC: Can Holistic Medicine Be Taught in Medical School American Holistic Medicine 1:40-45 1979.
13. Healey JM: Liability and Team care. Proceedings: Sixth Annual

Interdisciplinary Health Team Care Conference. September 19-21, 1984 Storrs, CT. School of Allied Health Professions, University of Connecticut.1985.

14. Pellegrino ED: What is A Profession? Journal of Allied Health 12:168-176. (August 1983).

15. Matejski MP: Ethical Issues in the Health Care System.Journal of Allied Health:131-139 (May 1982).

16. Katz D, Kahn R: The Social Psychology of Organizations, 2 Edition. John Wiley and Sons, New York. Chapters 12 and 13. 1978.

17. Chisholm RF, Zeigenfuss JT: A Review of Applications of the Sociotechnical Systems Approach to Health Care Organizations. Journal of Applied Behavioral Science 22:315-327. 1986.

18. Pava C: Redesigning Sociotechnical Systems Design: Concepts and Methods for the 90"s. Journal of Applied Behavioral Science 22:201-221. 1986.

19. Passmore W, Petee J, Bastian R: Sociotechnical Systems in Health care: A Field Experiment.Journal of Applied Behavioral Science 22:329-339. 1986.

20. Ivey S,Brown K,Teske Y,Silverman D: A Model for Teaching About Interdisciplinary Practice in Health Care Settings, Journal of Allied Health 17:189-195. (August 1988).

21. Williams F: The Impact of Scientific Advances on Programs. Geriatric Education-New Knowledge, New Settinqs, New Curriculum Proceedings of A Conference. Bethesda,MD Bureau of Health Professions, HRSA, HHS.June 2-4, 1986.

22. Connelly T: Basic Educational Considerations for Interdisciplinary Education Development in Health Sciences. Journal of Allied Health 7:274-280. Fall, 1978.

23. Burian B: Independent Practice? What is the Appropriate level of Autonomy For Health care Practitioners? Journal of Allied Health 18. Special Issue .

24. Proceedings of the Conference. Access of Quality Care In Rehabilitation. Washington DC. October 1988. (in press)

CHAPTER 12

The Future of Physical Therapy in Hospital Settings

Jane S. Mathews, MPH, PT

The chapters of this book have laid the foundation for understanding current physical therapy issues and practices in the milieu of the health care system in the United States during the late 1980s. An integral part of all the information shared was the message that continued changes and adjustments must be made to keep physical therapy a viable practice and profession for the future. To discern the potential trajectories, in a general sense, that can be used in planning for the future, many past and present trends and societal patterns can be examined. Some of these already have been discussed in detail throughout this book. Nonetheless, a summation that identifies future directions and paints a global picture is of value at this point because it emphasizes the importance of the quality needed for current professional decision making and planning efforts.

My intent is to present scenarios as a means of demonstrating potential outcomes in the year 2020 AD related to current practices, first in the health care system and then in physical therapy in hospital settings. With no claims of being a prophet, I will rely on my in-depth personal review of trends, reports, and articles such as the one entitled "Health Agenda for the American People" published by the American Medical Association in February 1987. Although some of my descriptions may border on levity to get a point across, my observations are less than humorous.

Additionally, you may find some of my scenarios positive and others negative. I have no intent to project a "doomsday" perspective but to point out that any scenario may result from effective decisions, poor decisions, or from a failure to make certain decisions. All interpretations in that regard are left entirely to the readers' individual judgments.

Scenario I—The Health Care System

The year is 2020 AD, just a mere 32 years from 1988. Some physical therapists may be at the peak of their careers, others will be entering retirement, and at least a few will be pushing up daisies in the year 2020.

Those daisies will be growing around grave markers made of plastic. Because the effects of acid rain east of the Mississippi river became so severe by the year 2000, markings on the older headstones have eroded and become indistinguishable.

Additionally, environmental toxicity was not controlled by society soon enough or rigorously enough. As a result, the incidence and prevalence of severe developmental disabilities, mental retardation, and learning disorders have increased by 2000% since the 1980s. The uncontrolled use of pesticides and food additives, the poisoning of water supplies, and the exposure of pregnant women and infants to cigarette smoke all have created major health problems.

The ground water pollution levels on Long Island, for example, are now so great that governmental agencies recommend that no children or pregnant women live there without using bottled water supplies. Additionally, in 2020 there is a nationwide warning that no children or pregnant women are safe from the effects of toxins if they live within three miles of a major thruway. Do you recall that there used to be major duck and potation producing industries on Long Island? It is sad to observe that both industries long since have become obliterated because of environmental toxins.

The numbers of persons with chronic mental illness have increased by 1,000% nationwide. During the past 32 years, our society continued to ignore this health problem, and, as more and more of these individuals remain untreated, they are turning in growing numbers to the streets and to crime. This change has greatly eroded the quality of life in our large cities, particularly those located in warmer climates. The state of Arizona, for example, which in 1988 had identified 9,000 citizens with this problem, now in 2020 has 90,000 citizens with chronic mental health problems; most of those remain without access to treatment.

Most of the small and medium-sized community hospitals as we knew them in the 1980s have closed long since. They could not survive financially the intensive competition for patients who from the early 1980s on were treated more and more in outpatient settings. Some old-timers remember how, after the advent of prospective payment systems in 1983, many of these hospitals joined the marketing bandwagon to the point where they were offering free appendectomies with every coronary bypass procedure and monthly "fire sales" in their sports medicine clinics. Those attempts to survive financially proved to be frantic and futile, and many hospitals did not survive. As a point of interest, the physical facilities of those closed hospitals now are being used as day care centers for infants, children, and the elderly.

As was projected in the 1980s, about 25% of the US population now is over 65 years of age, and this constituency has immense political power. One former politician who had opposed health care changes now is 111 years of age; he finally has evidenced concern with the health and welfare of the elderly. He functions as the advocate for this group, from his computer terminal at his ranch. He also is strongly opposed to a new mandatory euthanasia law that automatically applies to any citizens who have reached their 100th birthday.

Medical technology, such as miracle drugs, refined microsurgery techniques, and those marvelous new, computerized life support machines, now is able to fix almost anything broken or dysfunction in human body systems. The irony is that few people can pay for it. You see, since the turn of the 21st Century, the rationing of health care has become a grim reality. As early as the year 2013, organ transplants were reserved for only the very young or the very rich. Even young adults in their early 30s now are denied transplants as a result of the sheer cost of the care and the shrinking supply of healthy organs.

Health care rationing also has had some very positive outcomes. In the past three decades, citizens have assumed full responsibility for their personal health behaviors to an extent that far exceeds our wildest expectations at the height of the fitness craze in the late 1980s. From early childhood, citizens learn to monitor various aspects of their body systems through a small, computerized device that is worn on the wrist and is similar to a digital watch. When a system signals a variation from healthy norms, the device signals immediate action to be taken. Necessity indeed is the mother of intervention!

Acquired immunological deficiency remains a major health problem in terms of vast incidence and prevalence. Back in the 1980s, a virus related to causation was identified and a cure subsequently was developed in 1993. Unfortunately, but as predicted by a maverick biomedical researcher at the University of California in 1988, seven new strains developed; to date, no effective cures have been identified for any of those new strains.

One final observation can be made about the health care system of 2020 AD. The delivery of all types of health care services now is controlled largely by eight to ten megacorporations with a multiplicity of joint ventures, all of which are classified as "managed health care systems."

Few health maintenance organizations remain because their enrollments were predicated initially on primary populations of employed adults. As demographic shifts in the population occurred and an increasing proportion of the population was composed of the elderly, the health maintenance organizations lost their financial base and no longer were viable. Regardless of the disappearance of these organizations as we knew them when they were initiated, certain aspects have reached fruition in 2020. That is, the fact that the managements of the existing megacorporations now are exercising control over all decisions regarding the types of services delivered; where, when, and how frequently those services are delivered; and which types of providers will deliver the service. Providers of service now essentially have no say at all in the present system. We saw the beginnings of this over 33 years ago in the 1980s, but it was hard to believe. Perhaps we, as physical therapists, should have invested a stronger effort to substantiate our therapeutic interventions in order to retain a measure of credibility in the decision making about physical therapy services.

In summary, the characteristics of the health industry in 2020 are changed markedly from those of the 1980s. The severe rationing of health care services has greatly reduced the number of surgical interventions that formerly were a major source for hospital admissions. Now there are only half the number of hospitals as in the 1980s, and these primarily are large, tertiary care, teaching, medical centers in urban areas. Major health problems include AIDS, chronic mental illness, and various types of neurological dysfunction associated with the effects of environmental toxins. Managed health care systems prevail and literally control access to services in all types of settings through their predominance.

Scenario II—Physical Therapy in the Hospital Setting

Given the context of major characteristics of the health care system in the year 2020 AD, now let us examine physical therapy in the remaining hospital settings and attempt to identify what changes have occurred, if any.

First, I note that now in 2020 very few physical therapists are practicing in hospital settings. Those that remain in hospitals are all board certified in one or more of the now fifteen approved specialization areas. This situation has a complex etiology, so I will mention only a few of the major contributing factors.

Some of you may recall that in 1987 the House of Delegates of the American Physical Therapy Association passed a motion that enabled the APTA to collaborate with the American Hospital Association in a project designed to address the then apparent shortage of physical therapists in hospital settings. I was concerned at the outset because it did not appear that the concept of "shortage" had been defined adequately. Without a clear and mutually agreed-upon definition between the APTA and AHA, any outcomes of data gathering were compromised at the outset.

The AHA, for example, tended to define shortage only in terms of numbers (ie, numbers of vacant positions, numbers of new graduates each year, and numbers of practitioners lost through attrition from the profession). No real attention was given to an examination of the effectiveness of existing physical therapy delivery systems in hospitals, particularly the aspect pertaining to personnel utilization. At that time in my own consultation experiences in hospital settings, I repeatedly had observed personnel utilization patterns in physical therapy departments that not only suggested inefficiency but also appeared to be preordained to create problems with recruitment and retention. I, for example, observed many departments that were top heavy with licensed physical therapists but had insufficient numbers of supportive personnel such as physical therapist assistants and aides. That situation inevitably meant that physical therapists frequently were engaged in activities that could and should have been delegated to supportive personnel. I also observed in those hospitals that in certain other medical or surgical departments patients who required the expertise of physical therapists were going untreated because the physical therapy departments professed lack of sufficient manpower.

Beginning in the late 1970s, even newly graduated physical therapists started seeking practice environments other than hospital settings. This change appeared to be due mainly to practice conditions that tended to restrict the decision-making autonomy of physical therapists and failed to utilize the level of judgment and decision-making for which they had been educated. I personally suspect that the frustration of those new graduates was initiated during their clinical education experiences in hospitals as students. In fact, many students had expressed to me that their clinical experiences in those settings motivated them to identify hospitals as settings in which they did not wish to practice.

I also note that few physical therapists who are in the 2020 AD hospital settings are there under arrangements quite different from those back in the 1980s. Most are in hospitals on staff appointments through contractual agreements similar to medical staff appointments of yesteryear. Those physical therapists who did not pursue or who failed to meet the requirements for formal board certification for advanced competence in a specialization now are confined by regulatory agencies to certain institutional settings. With their mobility so restricted, many of those practitioners long since have left the profession and have switched to other career pursuits. This situation also has contributed to the decreased number of physical therapists in hospital settings.

I recall that back in the 1980s many physical therapists were concerned that only physical therapist assistants eventually would be practicing in hospital settings. That notion generated no small amount of fear, but my perception was contrary to that. As prospective payment was introduced in 1983 and patient lengths of stay were decreased significantly, it seemed to me that just the opposite would occur (ie, hospitals would require physical therapists with extensive expertise who would be equipped to make rapid and accurate patient care judgments). In the year 2020, the latter appears to have been the case.

It also is astonishing to observe that as physical therapy assessment and intervention technology became increasingly sophisticated through computerization, the therapy equipment and other devices became so small in size and so inexpensive that even hospital departments now can maintain state-of-the-art technology. That was not the case back in the 1980s when many hospital departments could not obtain the capital equipment funds to remain on he cusp of contemporary technology. This, in turn, may relate to another change that I observe in 2020.

Third-party payers, both public and private, now reimburse only for those physical therapy interventions that scientifically are documented as being effective in achieving specified functional outcomes within predictable time limits. The advancements in technology have enabled physical therapists to become far more precise and predictive and, in some ways, may account for the fact that physical therapy still has some services in the remaining hospital settings.

Additionally, I am pleased to observe the progress made in developing systems to monitor the quality of physical therapy services in hospitals and in other delivery settings. You may recall that physical therapists exercised passive resistance against such systems for many years and preferred that they remain voluntary. Thanks to third-party payer requirements and physical therapists' advancement in research over the past three decades, measures are now in place to make such systems effective and fair.

I also see some changes in relation to education, clinical education, and staff development in hospital settings. In 2020, 75% of the physical therapists available in hospital settings have been prepared in entry-level doctoral programs. They now receive their major clinical education in a residency model, similar to that initially used by medicine. Although the students still have clinical correlation experiences interwoven with their academic sequence of study, they must target specialty directions prior to graduation. There now is a nationwide, computerized residency-matching system in which students register in their final year of the entry-level program. They enter their residencies following completion of all degree requirements and obtainment of licensure.

Staff development in hospitals now is far more decentralized than it was in the 1980s. At that time, there was an abundance of continuing education programs that were highly expensive and that had no quality control monitoring. In those days, hospitals were in a financial struggle, and physical therapy departments seldom had significant budgetary allocations for continuing education. Furthermore, many colleagues frequently expressed their frustration after attendance at a continuing education course that did not meet their expectations (ie, in accordance with promises of the brochure).

Several events served to change this system. First, by 1992 the APTA recognized that it had a major responsibility for developing a system for monitoring the quality of all continuing education offerings, which included explicit criteria. Based on the criteria, the APTA now publishes periodic ratings of all offerings so that potential participants have a clear picture of the benefits and limitations of continuing education programs in which they invest. Second, hospital setting staff development now is predicated on a modified model. Formerly, in addition to inservice education, hospital physical therapy departments relied heavily on sending staff to external continuing education programs whenever resources would permit. The department personnel have recognized since that it is far more cost-effective to identify specific needs of staff development in relation to the clientele served by their institutions; they now bring the needed educational expertise to the department. This means that a much larger proportion of staff can benefit from the development opportunity at a lower cost in the long-run to the institution.

In the year 2020 productivity of physical therapy services in hospitals is an even greater priority than it was following the initiation of prospective payment in 1983. The hospitals that have survived financially have had the benefit of physical therapy department administrators who know how to measure productivity and how to justify department program development based on a balance between increased productivity projections and quality assurance. In fact, our entry-level education programs now are doing a much better job in preparing graduates to cope with the business of physical therapy as well as with preparation for client therapeutic interventions.

In 1988, some twenty-one states had obtained direct access legislation, but educational programs and practice settings then had not yet understood the magnitude of the implications of that legislation.

From the time the goal of postbaccalaureate degree entry-level education was established by the APTA House of Delegates in 1979, there was a justifiable reason for keeping the issues of direct access and educational preparation separate. The need for consciously planned linkages became apparent, however, as more and more states achieved direct access privileges and more and more educational programs made the transition to the postbaccalaureate degree.

Initially, the issues were separated because the profession believed that it should not take a stance that would imply that those therapists prepared in undergraduate programs were somehow incapable of functioning in a direct access mode. When it became clear that direct access legislation was being accepted, however, the APTA recognized the responsibility and obligation to foster linkages, (ie, linkages that would be designed to prepare entry-level program graduates to function even more effectively in direct access practice modes). Fortunately, the necessity for the linkage became apparent in the early 1990s and physical therapy educational programs began to respond accordingly.

There are at least two somewhat sad observations I must make about physical therapy in hospital settings in 2020. Therapists in general now have a client population consisting primarily of essentially well persons who receive interventions targeted to health promotion, fitness, and primary and secondary prevention of musculoskeletal dysfunction. I do not criticize that because it certainly took us a long time to get involved in health promotion and prevention activities.

Unfortunately, physical therapists no longer have a prominent role in the care of geriatric clients. Despite the population demographic shift predictions and the fact that nearly half of the physical therapists' clientele in 1988 was age 55 or over, the profession failed to give sufficient attention to providing the knowledge and skills needed to be responsive to the unique needs of the elderly. Also, it became very clear back in the 1980s that an increasing number of new physical therapy graduates appeared to prefer practice in orthopedic or sports injury settings, and few opted for geriatric service settings, which included hospitals. Sadly for the profession, but perhaps fortunate for the elderly, there were numerous other types of providers ready and willing to offer services in the geriatric arena, which in effect was lost by default.

As for the client population with chronic mental illness, the physical therapy profession never had major involvement. Although a small number of therapists practiced in psychiatric settings, they tended to respond primarily to the referrals of residents on a post-facto basis (ie, those residents with psychiatric problems who had sustained cerebrovascular accidents, fractures, or other pathological conditions). Few physical therapists recognized early enough that they could have had a major role in mental health, particularly in wellness programs targeted to maintenance of function and mobility. Given the extensive population of those with chronic mental illness in 2020, that indeed appears to be an unfortunately missed opportunity.

One final observation I wish to make that relates to physical therapy in hospital settings in the year 2020 AD pertains to the development of a common nomenclature or taxonomy.

As early as 1987, the APTA Committee on Practice identified the need for a manual on measurement similar to that published for many years by the American Psychology Association. That action was a beginning, but not enough. With the increasing emphasis on the rationing of health care and the decrease in lengths of hospital stays, it became increasingly important for physical therapists in all types of service settings to avoid activities that constituted redundancy or were conducive to patients-clients "falling through the cracks: of the health care system. One of best mechanisms identified by the turn of the 21st Century was that of developing systems of assessment and measurement used in all physical therapy service settings.

This system required the development of a common nomenclature, particularly in outcome functional assessment instruments, that could be used validly and reliably by any physical therapy service on referral of clients from hospital settings. Therapists in hospital settings had to take the lead in this movement to insure that clients, or their third-party payers, were not disadvantaged by the phenomenon of "repeating the wheel" as clients moved through a community health service delivery system.

Summary

If one reviews the history of the physical therapy profession, it becomes clear that practice in hospital settings has been and remains in part the cornerstone of physical therapy practice and education. Whether that remains to be the case in the future is subject to question. The APTA Membership Survey of 1987 indicates that about 42% of the sample respondents practice in hospital settings; therefore, hospital-based practitioners theoretically still have the potential to wield a mighty influence on the future. That influence of the future, however, will take a degree of leadership and responsiveness on the part of our hospital physical therapists that has not yet been evident.

Physical therapy practice in all settings, including hospitals, is undergoing change. How we, as physical therapists, do or do not develop capabilities for responding to that change in ways that pose the greatest benefits for our patient-client populations may hold the key to the nature of our professional role and functions in the next century. The professional practice in hospitals and in other service settings for physical therapists is being shaped right now. I firmly believe that our decisions now, as a profession and as a professional association, can shape the future. I also submit that the decision we fail to make or prefer to avoid today also will have an impact on our future as a profession practicing within or external to hospital settings.

Appendix

Professionalism in Physical Therapy

During the past few years, Jane Mathews, President of the APTA, has delivered a number of presentations focusing on professionalism to students of physical therapy and other health disciplines at graduations, conclaves, component meetings and additional occasions. The following timely advice--applicable to today's physical therapists as well as tomorrow's --is adapted from this series of presentations.

Professionalism. How do we as physical therapists define this word that has generated so much interest and discussion in our ranks?

Dictionary definitions give us little help. *The American Heritage Dictionary* defines professionalism as "...professional status, methods, character, or standards." According to *The Merriam-Webster Dictionary* it's: "...the conduct, aims, or qualities that mark a profession or a professional person."

But no clues are provided as to the kinds of "conduct, aims, or qualities" that are desirable.

So we must ask ourselves: What behaviors characterize professionalism in physical therapy?

I offer to you my personal perspective of physical therapy professionalism. The following "laundry list," which is based on my own experience and value systems, describes the behaviors and characteristics I believe mark the true physical therapy professional.

Full Accountability

The physical therapist professional accepts full accountability for her/his decisions and behaviors.

The development of professional accountability begins during the initial professional education. In your student years, you are accountable to your goals about pursuing a career in physical therapy. It means taking self-responsibility for learning.

Program faculty are there to facilitate that learning via the experiences they design, the materials they make available, and whatever insight or wisdom from their own experiences they can provide.

What students do with all that is entirely an individual responsibility.

Accountability at the student level also is manifested in other ways, such as getting to classes on time; being conscientious about client treatment schedules and meetings in the clinical education settings; and by completing assignments by the designated deadlines.

Excuses or blaming behaviors do not reflect professionalism.

The need for accountability tends to expand when one enters practice as acredentialed physical therapist.

You are still fully accountable to yourself and your clients, but now you hold an additional accountability to society and to your profession.

Remember that every action or behavior you adopt reflects the profession and shapes society's perceptions of physical therapy and physical therapists.

Lifelong Career Commitment

Physical therapy is not a "sometime" type of career. A lifelong career commitment does not necessarily mean continuous practice until you check into that great KIN-COM[fi]in the sky. But it does mean continuous commitment via the nature of your involvement.

You do not "work" in physical therapy or hold an 8:30 to 5:00 "job." As a physical therapist, you engage in professional practice that does not always guarantee specific hours or clear-cut schedules.

Several years ago, I was saddened by the comments from a student from another school who was taking the sophomore introductory physical therapy course at Boston University. The student initially had planned a career in medicine but, as she put it, she was exploring physical therapy because she thought it would be "less demanding."

Anyone entertaining that fantasy is headed for great disillusionment!

For a variety of reasons, both males and females may have to drop out of direct patient care for a period of time, e.g., to attend graduate school to raise families, to pursue other interests.

In such circumstances, however, you can still remain actively engaged in physical therapy by your community activity, your professional association involvement, and by keeping current on the trends and issues within PT and the health industry in general.

Commitment to LifeLong Learning

The physical therapist has a commitment to lifelong learning and professional development.

The committed physical therapist clearly understands that the initial professional education program is merely the basic foundation for a lifetime of learning.

Consider as an analogy for this the construction of a house. Your basic professional education represents merely the foundation consisting of the exterior and unfinished walls. You must add the windows, doors, trim, and all the other details through continued learning of both a formal and informal nature.

The quest for knowledge is infinite. Continuing professional development is required to remain at the cusp of physical therapy knowledge and skills. Your commitment to lifelong learning and professional development will best enhance the quality of services you provide to your clients.

Highest Ethical/Moral Standards

Our contemporary health care system is plagued with an ever-increasing number of complex ethical dilemmas.

To be ethical means that you make your practice decisions in accordance with the accepted principles of right and wrong that govern the conduct of your profession. Having made that admonition, I confess that the saying is far easier than the doing.

The bottom line in the resolution of any ethical or moral dilemma is *your* individual conscience.

A prime example is the current ethical dilemma among health care professionals about treating patients with AIDS.

My personal bottom line suggests that there *is* no dilemma. In other words, if any individual can benefit from my services, I am prepared to provide those services.

I acknowledge that not all of my professional colleagues share my perspective. The point is, that in any such dilemmas, you stand alone in making the ethical judgments according to *your* **value systems and** *your* **conscience.**

Value for Objectivity

A physical therapy professional evidences a value for objectivity in practice decisions and behaviors.

As a physical therapist, you are a health scientist. This fact should be reflected in both the process and outcomes of your decisions. A health scientist is prepared to provide rationales for every practice decision and can articulate these rationales to others.

A health scientist avoids the seduction of faddism or cultism in regard to popular treatment interventions or equipment.

A health scientist however, will be open-minded, will know how to research the literature and will weigh the evidence that documents the efficacy, or lack thereof, of a method, procedure, or modality.

Because you value objectivity, when you are seeking information on how to solve a problem presented by a client, you know how to conduct library research, how to seek consultation from peers with expertise, and how to use the numerous resource networks available within your chapter or national APTA office.

If you choose to be a full-time clinician, striving for excellence and desiring to make objective clinical decisions that enable effective and efficient treatment for your clients, you will never be inclined to say: "I don't have time to be involved in research because I'm here to treat patients."

If you're a full-time clinician, your opportunities to participate in basic or applied experimental research projects may indeed be limited. But you can create such opportunities and you can most certainly assist and facilitate research conducted by your colleagues.

Most important, you'll remember that every clinician has the opportunity for library research at his or her disposal. And your clients will benefit if you take advantage of such resources.

Skilled at Self-Criticism

If you evidence a value for objectivity, you will have the capability to be self-critical. Self-criticism relates to a range of activity including therapeutic interventions, knowledge, skills, interpersonal behaviors, and so on.

If you reach a point in your career when you think you have "all the answers," that may be just the time to indulge in introspection and self-criticism.

If you are self-critical, you will know how to solicit constructive feedback and how to give it. The skills needed to do this may not have been emphasized in your basic preparation program; but I see these skills as being just as important as clinical competence.

Self-criticism requires, for example, effective listening and responding skills; conflict resolution skills; a clear understanding of your personal styles of interaction and how these impact on others.

If your professional education curriculum didn't provide an opportunity to develop and/or refine these skills, then I strongly recommend you seek ways to obtain them in your continuing education.

Comfortable With Ambiguities

Ambiguities are a part of our profession and our professional practice.

At this stage in our evolution as a profession, physical therapy is far more an art than a science. We have multiple methods available to approach the same client problem and, as individuals, we have to choose the most appropriate method for the client at hand.

Whether you are a student or a credentialed practitioner, if you are still seeking "the one best way" to solve a particular client treatment problem, you're ripe for great frustration and unhappiness.

According to the literature, students have a tendency to view clinical supervisors as their primary role models. But what if the role model is advocating a method or intervention that has long since been obsolete? Sometimes academic faculty will promulgate *their* preferred method as "the one best way." In such cases, beware.

Remember that there may not be a "one best way," and your best course of action is research the literature to identify the intervention that has the best substantiation.

Understands the Business Aspects

The physical therapy professional places priority on clients' needs while still recognizing the business aspect of physical therapy.

The delivery of PT services includes a business aspect, regardless of the setting in which that delivery occurs.

You don't have to practice in a private setting to know you need to understand the business of PT.

PT practice has many business concerns. These concerns include reimbursement, personnel and staffing, marketing of services and service systems, financial planning and management, and many others.

Even as a salaried staff PT in a hospital department setting, you have a responsibility to develop an understanding of these business concerns--*if* you are truly interested in providing qualitative, cost-effective services to clients in need.

Developing and understanding of the business aspects of physical therapy does not mean that we are any less concerned about our clients and the quality of care they receive. Absolutely nothing is wrong with acknowledging that we, as physical therapists, are business persons as well as health care professionals.

The better the business relationships we establish, the better we will be able to provide quality services to our clients. The aspect of business and service to clients are highly compatible.

The relationship becomes distorted only when greed and avarice in relation to the business aspect take priority over client needs. And that can occur in *any* type of service delivery setting.

As professionals, we have to exercise the integrity and courage to ensure that we discourage the conditions that lead to such distortions. One way is to avoid practice environments in which your professional judgment as to whether a client does or does not need service is bypassed.

A classic example is the settings that benefit financially from a closed system of referrals and in which physical therapists do not have the final judgment as to access *to* treatment or termination *of* treatment.

Closed systems in any form place the client population at risk, and professionalism means being able to identify those circumstances to the extent that you avoid allowing yourself, your clients, or your profession to be subject to exploitation.

Ability to Articulate

As a physical therapy professional, you are able to articulate the philosophy and functions of your profession.

Articulation means not only the verbal translation or interpretation, but that which we also try to articulate in writing through documentation on the client record.

A recent General Accounting Office report on rehabilitation services indicated that more than 90 percent of the records in the report sampling did not contain adequate documentation for reimbursement.

Documentation in the client's record is one of the major ways we communicate our professional role and functions to others. In the instance cited, the documentation inadequacy related to Medicare beneficiaries. Unfortunately, that inadequacy extends to all other types of clientele and seems to be a problem nationwide.

If as physical therapists, we indeed have interventions that can benefit and improve the function of clients, we should be able to document and communicate that.

Respect Other Health Professionals

In the universe of health care, physical therapy is but a tiny planet. We do indeed have unique contributions to make to clients in their attempts to achieve optimal function, but, physical therapists are not the end-all or be-all of the health industry, nor are we the end-all or be-all in relation to client needs and services.

We cannot respect the unique aspects of other health care colleagues unless we make it a point to learn about their educational backgrounds, their roles and functions, and their philosophies and values.

We have an obligation to expand our knowledge in regard to every colleague with whom we interact in the provision of health care services.

An Advocacy Role

The physical therapy professional remains cognizant of, and is an advocate for, the ethnocultural groups in our society who have been disenfranchised (historically) on a consistent basis.

We have a special responsibility to be an advocate for populations in need of our services and for causes related to improving the *social* health of our society.

This advocacy role *must* be visible, articulate, and continuing.

Active in Professional Association

A physical therapy professional is actively engaged in the activities and affairs of the professional association (APTA) at all levels.

Please note that the key words are "actively engaged." Merely paying dues for an active membership category is insufficient.

The APTA House of Delegates (some 400-plus of your colleagues from around the country) make decisions that affect you.

If you do not become actively engaged at the district, chapter, section, or national levels via appointed or elected positions, you are essentially forfeiting the right to express your ideas and opinions.

Unfortunately, many of our dues-paying colleagues forfeit their rights by never attending Association meetings at any level.

Yet, they often complain vociferously about things "APTA" did or did not do, thus evidencing a lack of understanding that major policy decisions of the Association originate in the House of Delegates--a representative body selected by members at the component level.

Such decisions have included the transition to postbaccalaureate degree entry-level professional education programming by 1990, positions on issues such as referral-for-profit and direct access legislation, the creation of the formal board specialization processes to recognize advanced competence in six specialty areas, and so on.

Personally, I have never felt that merits of APTA membership can be argued on the basis of "benefits" received, e.g., publications, regulatory activities, member services.

I belong to APTA and remain actively engaged merely because I value the opportunity to express my opinions and for whatever small part those opinions play in the advancement of the profession.

A Balanced Personal Lifestyle

A physical therapist maintains and protects a balanced lifestyle.

Regardless of the behavioral burdens I may have imposed in all of the above, a person who demonstrates professional behaviors is not a person who lives in a thimble.

It is necessary to develop and maintain a broad-based lifestyle of personal interests relating to your leisure time, family, and interests. You will attempt to broaden your horizons through travel and reading, and you won't limit your social interactions only to those within or related to your profession.

For your personal mental health and well-being, you will maintain your interests in current events, including political activity.

Believe me, there *is* a life beyond physical therapy, and the colleagues I know and consider to be most highly imbued with professionalism protect that life rigorously!

The Infinite Challenge

I am aware that my "laundry list" of behaviors characterizing a true professional presents a heavy burden and an infinite challenge.

Our educational preparation and our experiences to date have prepared us for the challenge.

The bottom-line question for each of us to ask ourselves is: *Am I willing to face that challenge?*

Index

(HMOs), 94, 109, 111-117, 150
development of, 149
federally qualified vs. non-federally
qualified, 115
growth and acceptance of, 123
models of, 115-116
provider risks in, 123-124
vs. indemnity plan, 114
Health plans, prepaid, 90
HMO Assistance Act, 111, 113
Hospital information systems, 135-136
Hospitals
employment of physical therapists
and assistants, 72, 78
future of physical therapy in,
159-166
House calendar, 101
House of Representatives
consideration of legislation, 101-102
resolution of differing legislative
version from Senate, 102-103
Human engineering, 139
Humanitarianism, 13
Indemnity plans, 109-110, 114
Independent health plans, 94
Independent Practice, 23. See also
Direct access
Independent practice association
model, for HMOs, 115
Information management
in clinical decision analysis, 139-140
computerized medical advances,
128-129
education and, 132-135
in exercise and adaptive equipment
areas, 138-139
financial accounting systems,
135-136
growth stages of, 127-128
patient monitoring systems,
128-129
practice management and, 135
research and, 129-132
Information services for clinical
setting, 137-138
Institutions, educational
admissions, independent control
of, 17
discontinuance of physical therapy
education programs, 6
enrollment in, 19, 82
establishment of physical therapy
education programs, 6

faculty. See Faculty
financial reimbursement, 84
financial struggles of, 81-82
increasing class size of, 18
mission of, 5-6
organizational structure of, 6-7
philosophy and rationale of
programs, 82
processing of applications, 19
recognition of physical therapy
profession, 7
Interdisciplinary practice
basis of, 146
building teams for, 153-154
collaboration and, 145, 146
consumer involvement and,
150-151
future of, 154-155
health policy development and,
147-148
meeting technological demands,
153
need for, 148
organization of, 146-147
preparation for, 154
professional association, action
agenda for, 155-156
reality of current environment and,
148-150
status and independence for
physical therapy and, 151-153
value of, 145
Internship opportunities, 87
Joint resolution, 99-100
Joint venture, 43
Kaiser Permanent, 111
Legislation. See also specific
legislation
calendars, 101
changes, professional education
and, 79-80
committee action on, 100-101
consent measures, 101
direct access, 33
federal deficit and, 98
house consideration, 101-102
impact on scope and quality of
service, 98
introduction of, 99-100
Presidential action, 103-108
professional change and, 12
providers of service, impact on, 98
referral to committee, 100

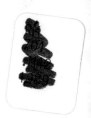

DATE DUE

Reserve
Peters
Fall 1997